D1562437

ETHICS IN ONCOLOGY NURSING

Edited by

Jeanne M. Erickson, PhD, RN, AOCN®
Kate Payne, JD, RN, NC-BC

Oncology Nursing Society
Pittsburgh, Pennsylvania

ONS Publications Department
Publisher and Director of Publications: William A. Tony, BA, CQIA
Managing Editor: Lisa M. George, BA
Assistant Managing Editor: Amy Nicoletti, BA, JD
Acquisitions Editor: John Zaphyr, BA, MEd
Copy Editors: Vanessa Kattouf, BA, Andrew Petyak, BA
Graphic Designer: Dany Sjoen
Editorial Assistant: Judy Holmes

Library of Congress Cataloging-in-Publication Data

Names: Erickson, Jeanne M., editor. | Payne, Kate (Clinical ethicist),
    editor. | Oncology Nursing Society, issuing body.
Title: Ethics in oncology nursing / edited by Jeanne M. Erickson, Kate Payne.
Description: Pittsburgh, Pennsylvania : Oncology Nursing Society, [2016] |
    Includes bibliographical references and index.
Identifiers: LCCN 2015049031 | ISBN 9781935864561
Subjects: | MESH: Oncology Nursing--ethics
Classification: LCC RC263 | NLM WY 156 | DDC 174.2/96994--dc23 LC record available at
    http://lccn.loc.gov/2015049031

Publisher's Note

This book is published by the Oncology Nursing Society (ONS). ONS neither represents nor guarantees that the practices described herein will, if followed, ensure safe and effective patient care. The recommendations contained in this book reflect ONS's judgment regarding the state of general knowledge and practice in the field as of the date of publication. The recommendations may not be appropriate for use in all circumstances. Those who use this book should make their own determinations regarding specific safe and appropriate patient care practices, taking into account the personnel, equipment, and practices available at the hospital or other facility at which they are located. The editors and publisher cannot be held responsible for any liability incurred as a consequence from the use or application of any of the contents of this book. Figures and tables are used as examples only. They are not meant to be all-inclusive, nor do they represent endorsement of any particular institution by ONS. Mention of specific products and opinions related to those products do not indicate or imply endorsement by ONS. Websites mentioned are provided for information only; the hosts are responsible for their own content and availability. Unless otherwise indicated, dollar amounts reflect U.S. dollars.

ONS publications are originally published in English. Publishers wishing to translate ONS publications must contact ONS about licensing arrangements. ONS publications cannot be translated without obtaining written permission from ONS. (Individual tables and figures that are reprinted or adapted require additional permission from the original source.) Because translations from English may not always be accurate or precise, ONS disclaims any responsibility for inaccuracies in words or meaning that may occur as a result of the translation. Readers relying on precise information should check the original English version.

Printed in the United States of America

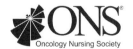

Innovation • Excellence • Advocacy

Contributors

Editors

Jeanne M. Erickson, PhD, RN, AOCN®
Assistant Professor
University of Wisconsin–Milwaukee
College of Nursing
Milwaukee, Wisconsin

Kate Payne, JD, RN, NC-BC
Associate Professor of Nursing
Center for Biomedical Ethics and
Society
Vanderbilt University Medical Center
Nashville, Tennessee

Authors

Courtney Buratto, MSN, FNP-C, OCN®
Nurse Practitioner
Community Hospital Oncology Physicians
Indianapolis, Indiana
Chapter 9. Ethics Consultation and Education

Amy M. Haddad, PhD, RN
Director
Center for Health Policy and Ethics
Dr. C.C. and Mabel L. Criss Endowed
Chair in Health Sciences
Creighton University
Omaha, Nebraska
Chapter 1. Principles of Ethics

Cathy Campbell, PhD, RN
Associate Professor
University of Virginia School of Nursing
Charlottesville, Virginia
Chapter 3. Treatment Decision Making

Dany M. Hilaire, PhD, RN
PhD Student
University of Massachusetts
Boston, Massachusetts
Chapter 6. Communication and Ethics

Rose Ermete, RN, BSN, OCN®, CCRP
Quality Assurance Nurse Auditor
SWOG
Livonia, Michigan
Chapter 2. Medical Research and Clinical Trials

Karen Iseminger, PhD, ANP-BC, FNP
Professor of Nursing
Affiliated Faculty
Center of Aging and Community
University of Indianapolis
Ethics Consultant
St. Vincent Health
Indianapolis, Indiana
Chapter 9. Ethics Consultation and Education

Randy A. Jones, PhD, RN, FAAN
Associate Professor
Robert Wood Johnson Foundation Nurse
  Faculty Scholar Alumnus
University of Virginia School of Nursing
Charlottesville, Virginia
Chapter 3. Treatment Decision Making

Jessica Keim-Malpass, PhD, RN
Assistant Professor
University of Virginia School of Nursing
Charlottesville, Virginia
Chapter 5. Patient Advocacy

Melissa Kurtz, MSN, MA, RN
Nurse Clinician and PhD Student
Johns Hopkins University
Baltimore, Maryland
*Chapter 8. The Impact of Ethical
Conflict and Dilemmas on Nurses*

Dale Halsey Lea, MPH, RN, CGC
(at the time of writing)
Consultant, Public Health Genomics
Maine Genetics Program
Maine Department of Health and Hu-
  man Services
Augusta, Maine
Chapter 7. Genetics and Genomics

**Samuel G. Robbins, DNP, MTS,
  ANP-BC, ACHPN**
Assistant in Medicine
Vanderbilt University School of Medi-
  cine
Nashville, Tennessee
*Chapter 4. Palliative and End-of-Life
Care*

**Cynda Hylton Rushton, PhD, RN,
  FAAN**
Anne and George L. Bunting Professor
  of Clinical Ethics
Johns Hopkins University
Baltimore, Maryland
*Chapter 8. The Impact of Ethical
Conflict and Dilemmas on Nurses*

**Lisa Kennedy Sheldon, PhD, APRN-
  BC, AOCNP®, ANP-BC**
Associate Professor
College of Nursing and Health Sciences
University of Massachusetts
Boston, Massachusetts
Chapter 6. Communication and Ethics

Susan Storey, PhD, RN, AOCNS®
Assistant Scientist
Indiana University School of Nursing
Indianapolis, Indiana
*Chapter 9. Ethics Consultation and
Education*

Disclosure

Editors and authors of books and guidelines provided by the Oncology Nursing Society are expected to disclose to the readers any significant financial interest or other relationships with the manufacturer(s) of any commercial products.

A vested interest may be considered to exist if a contributor is affiliated with or has a financial interest in commercial organizations that may have a direct or indirect interest in the subject matter. A "financial interest" may include, but is not limited to, being a shareholder in the organization; being an employee of the commercial organization; serving on an organization's speakers bureau; or receiving research funding from the organization. An "affiliation" may be holding a position on an advisory board or some other role of benefit to the commercial organization. Vested interest statements appear in the front matter for each publication.

Contributors are expected to disclose any unlabeled or investigational use of products discussed in their content. This information is acknowledged solely for the information of the readers.

The contributors provided the following disclosure and vested interest information:
Jeanne M. Erickson, PhD, RN, AOCN®: Josiah Macy Foundation, University of Virginia School of Medicine, research funding

Kate Payne, JD, RN, NC-BC: St. Thomas West Hospital, University Community Health Services, Edge of the Map Consulting, employment or leadership position; Ethics Consultant Group, Sumner Regional Medical Center, Alive Hospice, consultant or advisory role; Belmont University, Northwest Organization of Nurse Executives, Faith Community Nursing, Salem Health, Bailey Manor and Senior Advantage, Tennessee Organization of Nurse Executives, honoraria

Amy M. Haddad, PhD, RN: American Society for Bioethics and Humanities, leadership position

Karen Iseminger, PhD, ANP-BC, FNP: NRG Oncology, consultant or advisory role; American Nurses Association Center for Ethics and Human Rights, leadership position

Jessica Keim-Malpass, PhD, RN: National Cancer Institute, research funding

Melissa Kurtz, MSN, MA, RN: Johns Hopkins Ethics Consultation Service, American Society for Bioethics and Humanities Nursing Affinity Group Advisory Council, *Medical Ethics Advisor* Newsletter, consultant or advisory role; National Institutes of Health, research funding; Johns Hopkins School of Nursing, other remuneration

Lisa Kennedy Sheldon, PhD, APRN-BC, AOCNP®, ANP-BC: Middle East Cancer Consortium, honoraria; National Cancer Institute, research funding

Contents WITHDRAWN

Preface

The idea for this book grew out of a conversation following a presentation at the 2011 Scripps Cancer Center Oncology Nurses Symposium. This presentation discussed ethical issues facing oncology nurses, specifically when medicine cannot save a patient. Discussion with conference participants, and later with Oncology Nursing Society (ONS) staff, highlighted the difficulty and prevalence of ethical issues that oncology nurses face each day.

Oncology care and treatment raise complex and often troubling issues for patients, families, and nurses. Sometimes, ethical principles and obligations are in conflict, which creates ethical dilemmas. Bioethics as a discipline seeks to help nurses and other healthcare professionals discern the right thing to do in the face of such conflict. Decisions often require consideration of multiple factors in addition to the patient's physical condition. Ethics helps to separate what is medically possible from what is beneficial for the patient and to set norms for proper patient research. Ethics also clarifies the reasons that we give for our choices and actions as nurses. Often, questions are about what we should do and why—not about what we can do.

Ethics also expands the influence of health care on caregivers. Nursing cannot be viewed as merely a job description, but rather as a series of relationships. Through these relationships, nurses become connected to their patients and vice versa. Ethics is embedded in these relationships, allowing nurses to understand their patients' needs. Ethical issues also are threaded through our relationships with peers and colleagues as well as our own families and loved ones.

Paying attention to ethics helps us to feel and do better as nurses. It helps us know that there is benefit, even when a patient's disease leads to an untimely death. It helps us remember that people are ends unto themselves, never a means. The primacy of patients and their inherent worth and dignity are at the heart of nursing. Nurses are guided by the commitment to value those cared for as well as other caregivers and themselves.

In addition to foundational content on ethics and ethical practice, chapters in this book address key areas in oncology nursing associated with ethical concerns. Each chapter is authored by an expert on the subject and structured with specific content on each topic, implications for practice, and application in a case study. The authors chose topics that commonly raise ethical issues for oncology nurses. References are included at the end of each chapter for further study and discovery.

We are grateful to every author who provided such thoughtful and provocative chapters. They were labors of love. We also are thankful for the staff at ONS, who were tireless in shepherding this project through to publication, especially to Lisa George, our managing editor, who is forever patient and kind. And bless our families and friends, who were and always are encouraging.

We hope this book serves to enhance your ethical knowledge and skills and your desire to dive into an ethical dilemma in service of your patients and practice.

CHAPTER 1

Principles of Ethics

Amy M. Haddad, PhD, RN

Introduction

What kinds of acts are right in oncology nursing practice? This basic yet complex question is commonly asked by nurses in oncology and other specialties to determine what they should do in a specific case or how the entire profession should act regarding interactions with patients, families, and colleagues. General ethical principles often are used as guides for right action. The first such contemporary example that proposed principles as guides in a health-related area was the Belmont Report (National Commission for the Protection of Human Subjects of Biomedical and Behavioral Research, 1979), which identified the principles of respect for persons, beneficence, and justice in human subjects research. In 1981, Beauchamp and Childress built on this work and applied it to health care in the first edition of their book *Principles of Biomedical Ethics*, now in its seventh edition (Beauchamp & Childress, 2012). They proposed four key principles: respect for autonomy, beneficence (the obligation to do good), nonmaleficence (the duty not to harm), and justice. Others in bioethics have suggested additional derivative principles, including veracity (the obligation to tell the truth), fidelity (the duty to keep promises), and avoidance of killing (Veatch, Haddad, & English, 2010).

Although helpful in illuminating shared values and important ethical norms in health care, the principlist approach to ethics is not without its problems and critics. For example, polarities and problems exist within the principles themselves, such as tensions between present versus future expressions of autonomy (Collopy, 1988) or disagreement regarding who is best suited to determine benefit (Childress, 1982). Conflicts can also arise between principles, such as when one is attempting to fulfill the demands of respect for autonomy, which can run counter to the health professional's obligation to avoid harm. Additionally, no one principle of the four is given primacy, so determining which principle carries the day in a specific case is difficult. Critics have noted that the universal, objective nature of principlism seems to ignore the specific context of an ethical action, which they consider to be an integral component of moral decision making and reflection (Clouser & Gert, 1990; Jecker & Reich, 1995). Even with these criticisms and problems, principlism is the most commonly used approach in healthcare settings and, therefore, is an important part of ethical deliberations.

The focus of this chapter is to provide an introduction to the contributions of ethical principles to oncology nursing practice as well as their limitations. Emphasis is placed on the word *introduction,* as the discipline of ethics is complicated and what may at first appear to be a clear application to practice often has hidden difficulties. A helpful metaphor for the discussion of principles and other components of ethics is to think about what happens when a flashlight shines in a darkened room. A flashlight highlights wherever its beam falls and obscures everything else in the room. The flashlight also causes us to see things in a different, heightened way than we would under normal lighting (Dougherty, Edwards, & Haddad, 1990).

Principles and other elements of ethics often work in a similar way. Principles can illuminate realities and relationships that we might not have noticed otherwise, but they can also de-emphasize other equally important components of ethics. To help provide a more complete picture of what is involved in ethics, the selected case study aims to not only highlight where traditional ethical principles are at play in oncology nursing practice but also to enhance understanding of ways to approach ethical concerns.

Basic Principles of Ethics

Ethics is the branch of philosophy that explores moral duty, values, and character. In effect, ethics involves the study of right and wrong, moral responsibilities of actors, individual/institutional/societal moral conduct, promises, rules, principles, and theories. The study of ethics can also involve the moral value of relationships and other contextual issues, such as power structures and sources of knowledge. Together, these constitute important concerns in contemporary ethics. As noted, there are several approaches to ethics, but the one that is most relevant to an exploration of ethical principles is normative ethics. "Normative ethics raises the question of what is right or what ought to be done in a situation that calls for a moral decision. It examines individual rights and obligations as well as the common good" (Davis, Aroskar, Liaschenko, & Drought, 1997, p. 2).

This chapter will examine the relationship of principles to ethical situations in oncology nursing. However, the moral life is more than merely making discrete decisions to do this or not do that but rather encompasses how people live and think about these matters and, perhaps more importantly, how people work with others to discern the course of action. Therefore, reflection and discussion about ethical actions is also necessary for a fuller understanding of what acts are right. How nurses live the practice of and think about oncology nursing is particularly important because of the often life-threatening and always life-altering nature of cancer. Even in cases where cancer becomes a chronic condition with years of remission and recurrence, the nature of a cancer diagnosis often places the oncology nurse in complex ethical situations.

A brief, overarching explanation of the principlism of Beauchamp and Childress (2012) in their now classic *Principles of Biomedical Ethics* is in order before turning to specific principles. Beauchamp and Childress (2012) proposed a methodology to resolve ethical problems that is universally applicable in healthcare settings. As described by Viafora (1999), "Principlism relies upon a core of fundamental principles—themselves based upon some general theory—to be applied to rules which function as action-guides" (p. 285).

Therefore, the principles serve as a framework, and health professionals provide the "facts" of the situation or case in question, which when fed into the framework should ideally provide answers or, at minimum, insight into morally correct options.

Principles are based on more general theories. It is helpful to distinguish which theories support which principles. By shining a light on the theory, one can see the differences between principles that are oriented to consequences of actions and those that assert that the rightness or wrongness of an act is inherent in the act itself. The theoretical approach to ethics that focuses on outcomes is often referred to as the *consequentialist view*. A consequentialist deems actions as morally correct when they promote good. In other words, one should choose the action that brings about the most good, or, if there is little chance for a good outcome, the action that yields the least harm. An example of consequentialism in health care is the Hippocratic tradition in medicine that is based on the promotion of good for patients to the exclusion of other goods (Edelstein, 1987). Emphasis on the primacy of patient benefit is also evident in the American Nurses Association's (ANA's) *Code of Ethics for Nurses*, which states, "The nurse's primary commitment is to the recipients of nursing and healthcare services—patient or client—whether individuals, families, groups, communities, or populations" (ANA, 2015, p. 5). There are, of course, more complicated theoretical models of consequentialism, but this basic definition will suffice for this introductory chapter. Principles that derive from a consequentialist perspective are beneficence and nonmaleficence, two of the foundational principles proposed by Beauchamp and Childress (2012). Even without a background in philosophy, almost all health professionals would acknowledge the duty or obligation to do good for patients and to avoid as much harm as possible. Although the two principles can, and some would argue should, be discussed separately, they often are intertwined in clinical practice. One distinction between the two principles is that nonmaleficence is an absolute moral duty in that one is always obligated to avoid harming others. The principle of beneficence, however, is almost an imperative in health care in that it implies that one should promote good but not to the same degree in every case. Beneficence, therefore, is a relative duty in that the obligation to do good for others is tempered by other factors, such as the relationship held by those involved.

Nonmaleficence

The obligation not to harm others would seem to take priority over most other ethical principles. Beauchamp and Childress (2012) noted the connection between the principle of nonmaleficence and beneficence but resisted the idea of a hierarchal ordering of the two principles. They proposed the following norms:

Nonmaleficence
1. One ought not to inflict evil or harm.
Beneficence
1. One ought to prevent evil or harm.
2. One ought to remove evil or harm.
3. One ought to do or promote good.

Each of the three principles of beneficence requires taking action by helping—preventing harm, removing harm, and promoting good—whereas nonmaleficence requires only intentionally refraining from actions that cause harm. Rules of nonmaleficence therefore take the form "Do not do X." (Beauchamp & Childress, 2012, p. 152)

Some rules, such as "Do not lie to a patient" or "Do not harm one patient to benefit another," conform to the aims of nonmaleficence. However, as with most clinical situations, the rule of not harming is not as clear when applied to clinical practice. For example, a patient with metastatic cancer develops a bowel obstruction that appears to be due to benign strictures from previous surgery. Surgical intervention is indicated to correct the bowel obstruction, but, given the patient's cancer stage and general physical condition, the treatment team is divided regarding whether surgery in this case is a benefit or a harm. As with any surgical procedure, there are inherent risks and, given the patient's health status, the long-term benefits from surgery seem small in comparison. The short-term benefits of surgery, though, may loom large for the patient because of the nausea and acute pain that accompany bowel obstruction. There are also immediate life-threatening implications, such as ischemia of the bowel, that could be weighed differently by the patient and the surgical team. Thus, defining harm in order to avoid it is a more nuanced task than it first appears. Clinical parameters, patient and health professional values, and the relative balance between harms and benefits all play a part in determining harm.

Beneficence

The duty to do good is a strong one in health care. Whether informed by a religious tradition or basic human concern for the well-being of others, the directive to "love thy neighbor" underlies the actions of health professionals. Although we may be called to "love one another" in the broadest sense, it is clear that our capacity to love is limited by many things, including lack of time, knowledge, or resources. So, beneficence, the duty to do good, is limited, and we must choose among limited options to determine where we can do the most good (Glaser, 1994).

In the delivery of oncology nursing care, all of the nurse's actions are directed toward the good of the patient in whatever way "good" is defined. Beneficence is demonstrated in the smallest of actions and interactions with the patient, from a comforting touch to attentive listening. In addition, the principle of beneficence requires respect for the wishes and choices of the patient or family because such choices reflect interpretation of the good or what is of benefit. The nurse also has a privileged perspective on decisions and outcomes because of advanced education and experience. In contrast, the patient may be at a disadvantage when making decisions because of lack of healthcare knowledge and the additional stressors of illness. This is where other ethical principles come into play, such as respect for autonomy and the derived principle of consent that bolsters the patient's ability to make informed decisions. Beyond ensuring that patients have adequate information to determine the good and bad outcomes of actions, there can be differences in how the good is interpreted. For example, pain management would seem to be an uncontested good in patient care. However, the experience of pain and pain tolerance is highly subjective. Some patients may insist on the complete elimination of pain, whereas others may tolerate more pain to maintain a greater degree of consciousness. Patients may attach religious or redemptive meaning to pain that will alter how they consider the benefits and harms of pain relief. What may seem like a straightforward "good" in oncology nursing (i.e., relieving pain) is complicated in clinical practice. Discerning benefit should be an ongoing, collaborative process between the patient and family and the nurse. Balancing goods and harms as a broader principle is sometimes referred to as *proportionality* and will be discussed later in this chapter.

Respect for Autonomy

Some principles are based on the inherent rightness or wrongness of an action rather than the consequences of the action. "These positions, collectively known as formalism or deontologism, hold that right- and wrong-making characteristics may be independent of consequences, that morality is a matter of duty rather than merely evaluating consequences" (Veatch et al., 2010, p. 11). The duty to respect autonomy is one of these principles. The concept of respect for autonomy is based on a more fundamental principle of respect for persons. Respect for persons requires that individuals treat each other with respect regardless of conditions such as status, age, race, decision-making capacity, and so on. People are obligated to respect others merely because they are human. People are not, however, obligated to respect any and all actions of others, which is an important distinction.

If people are duty-bound to respect others, it follows that people should also respect their ability to make choices about how they will live their lives. The most fundamental aspect of respect for autonomy is the notion of noninterference with others. In a world of strangers, this idea of leaving others free to carry out their daily lives and business makes sense. Noninterference in healthcare relationships, however, does not make as much sense because health professionals are essentially asked to "interfere" with deeply personal facets of a person's life in order to cure, heal, and comfort.

Where autonomy plays a larger role in healthcare interactions is respect for self-determination, or being one's own person and making decisions about one's own well-being. Autonomy reflects a person's ability to express needs and control decisions. Whenever a person is ill, autonomy can be threatened. Patients with cancer need to make decisions about many aspects of their care, including whether to pursue standard or experimental treatment, which requires a higher level of informed consent. Because no one is capable of being completely or fully autonomous, acceptance occurs along a range of substantially autonomous decision making in which a person has "enough" understanding, information, and freedom to come to a sound decision in a particular context (Beauchamp & Childress, 2012). The amount of understanding, information, and freedom will vary from person to person and within the same person over time because of illness or injury. Determining whether a decision or action is substantially autonomous is important because of the obligation to honor autonomous actions even if the decision could lead to harm.

Justice

The principle of justice addresses the proper distribution of benefits and burdens. The allocation of healthcare resources is an abiding problem in health care. Oncology nursing is no exception. Distribution of resources can occur on various levels, from societal to personal. Justice also embodies the ideal of fairness. When one thinks of what is fair or just in a situation, he or she usually thinks about claims between people and rules to help mediate such claims. Consider the following example: Three patients arrive at the same time for their chemotherapy treatment at an ambulatory oncology clinic. One patient has arrived early for her appointment because she wants to talk to the nurse about a list of side effects and possible homeopathic remedies. The second patient is very weak and seems somewhat short of breath. The third patient is here for his final round of treatment and currently has few complaints. The nurse notes that all the other clinic nurses are busy, so she cannot delegate to a peer. She must decide which patient will get her initial attention. In order to make such a decision, the nurse is relying on principles of justice. The nurse could decide to spend her time with the patient where her actions will do the most good. Or, she could decide to direct her attention to the patient in the greatest need. Determining the distribution of healthcare resources, whether they be nursing time, access to diagnostic tests, or expensive medication, is one of the most complicated ethical problems in health care today.

Three additional principles deserve mention because of their importance in clinical practice: truth telling, fidelity (promise keeping), and avoidance of killing. These three principles are duty-based in that the right-making characteristic of the principles are inherent in the principles themselves, not the consequences.

Truth Telling

The principle of veracity, or truth telling, requires that healthcare providers be honest in their interactions with patients. "Traditional ethics holds that it is simply wrong morally to lie to people, even if it is expedient to do so, even if a better outcome will come from the lie. According to this view, lying to people is morally wrong in that it shows lack of respect for them" (Veatch & Haddad, 2008, p. 102). Being honest with patients helps to build and maintain trusting relationships that are essential to the delivery of quality patient care. However, as with the other principles, telling the truth to a patient is not always viewed as the right thing to do. Although mainstream American culture holds honesty in high regard, other cultures do not. In fact, telling sick and dying people about their conditions, particularly in the case of terminal illness, can be seen as cruel and even harmful by certain ethnic and racial groups (Blackhall, Frank, Murphy, & Michel, 2001). The principle of truth telling is influenced, interpreted, and valued differently because of the backgrounds, education, and socioeconomic status of providers and patients.

Fidelity

Moral theologian Paul Ramsey maintained that the fundamental question in healthcare ethics relates to the principle of fidelity.

> We are born within covenants of life with life. By nature, choice, or need we live with our fellowmen in roles or relations. Therefore we must ask, what is the meaning of the *faithfulness* of one human being to another in every one of these relations? This is the ethical question. (Ramsey, 2002, p. xlv)

Fidelity is rooted in respect for persons and truth telling. Faithfulness to promises is important in relationships because it indicates the level of esteem held for one another and establishes trust. When a person makes a promise, he or she creates expectations of another. The person expects to rely on the promise and have a valid claim that it will be kept. When a nurse assures a patient that he or she will receive appropriate symptom management while undergoing chemotherapy, the message does not have meaning unless the nurse follows through on that promise when it is actually needed during treatment. Fidelity is also important in interactions with peers on the healthcare team. Generally, promises to peers are not explicit but are shown through actions that implicit promises are being kept regarding important aspects of working together, such as honesty, not taking advantage of each other, and demonstrating dependability to be there for help and assistance when needed.

Avoidance of Killing

Although the principle of nonmaleficence would seem to prohibit active killing, some ethicists have argued that the seriousness and finality of killing requires a separate principle that specifically recognizes the prohibition (Veatch, 1981). Active killing can be deemed wrong from consequentialist (great and irreversible harm occurs) and duty-based (violates autonomy) perspectives. However, there are instances when killing could be justified, such as during war or in self-defense. There are also instances in which a person could consent to killing, as is the case with assisted suicide or voluntary euthanasia. Even with consent and the backing of law, as is the case in the states of Montana, Washington, Oregon, Vermont, and California, traditional religious and secular ethics has held to a prohibition of killing, even for merciful reasons. Patient requests to hasten death occurred frequently enough in oncology nursing practice that the Oncology Nursing Society (ONS) developed a position statement on hastening death. In the position statement, ONS recognized the nurse's right "to refuse to be involved in the care of patients who choose hastened death as a course of action" in jurisdictions where it is legally sanctioned (ONS, 2010, p. 249). The position statement also indicates that as a professional organization, ONS does not support actions that hasten death. ANA (2013) held a similar view in its position statement on euthanasia, assisted suicide, and aid in dying. In 2011, the Hospice and Palliative Nurses Association (HPNA) issued a position, endorsed by ONS, that identified nurses' rights to "decide whether their own moral and ethical value system does or does not allow them to be involved in providing care to a patient who has made the choice to end his or her life through [assisted death]" (HPNA, 2011, p. 2).

Virtue and Care-Based Ethics

While principlism focuses on actions, the character of the actor and where the actor is situated are obscured. Once again, a brief overview of two other approaches to ethics, virtue and care-based, provides a fuller view of ethics. Virtue ethics spotlights moral character rather than actions, as the following summary description of the theory notes.

> Virtue ethics starts instead with the insight that our actions, by and large, are not isolated decisions that we make, but arise from our character, the deeper complement of typical patterns of behavior that we exhibit, and the values that we hold. These character traits are not static, but are shaped and re-shaped con-

tinually by the actions we choose, and our reflection on those actions and their meaning in our lives. (Fullam, 2006, para. 2)

The development of virtues is, therefore, a formative process that is shaped by many elements. Role models likely contributed to the person that each individual has become. Beyond personal virtues, one can also consider the virtues of the whole nursing profession. Consider which virtues are central to oncology nursing, such as compassion, competence, and courage, and how these virtues are supported and nurtured in clinical practice. Such virtues incline the nurse who possesses them to act in certain ways regardless of whether there is supporting knowledge about which ethical principle justifies the actions.

Care-based ethics is often associated with responsiveness to particular incidents rather than an objective moral view. The details matter in care-based ethics, as do relationships. Care-based ethics also recognizes a sort of kinship with others who share the human condition and all of its frailties. Such a view acknowledges that people are not all equally situated in life and that these differences in status and other aspects of life have moral meaning. Sometimes referred to as *mutuality*, another component of care-based ethics views relationships as processes that are negotiated and collaborative in which all involved parties participate, choose, and act (Storch, Rodney, & Starzomski, 2004). Finally, there is recognition of the role of emotions in care-based ethics that is lacking in the objective stance of principlism. The basic argument against emotions as a moral guide is that they are unreliable and changeable. Little (1996) presented a counterview of the role of emotions in ethics, noting that emotions can lead us to attend to the "particulars" in a situation that can be helpful in recognizing an individual's needs. Without this emotional connection, we could miss important information that distance obscures.

Thus, where one stands in relation to another is morally salient in care-based ethics, which aligns with many of the values of the nursing profession. Both virtue and care-based ethics provide another vision of ethics that draws attention to the moral agent, who he or she is as a person, and the specific circumstances and relationships in particular situations that also influence action and the priority of responsibilities.

Cases in Ethical Reflection

Rather than starting with abstract rules or theories, a clinical case is useful to illustrate the realities of healthcare practice. Arras (1994) presented a basic argument for the use of cases or narratives in ethical reflection: "I think all would agree that a complete story or history is a prerequisite to any responsible moral analysis. Before one can attempt to judge, one must understand, and the best way to understand is to tell a nuanced story" (p. 1004). The following case was selected for analysis because it does not specifically deal with a significant ethical issue, such as a life-or-death decision or the use of expensive or experimental therapy, but rather with a very pedestrian intervention—that is, whether or not to turn a patient who is in bed. Because ethical issues sometimes get lost in urgent, high-technology cases, a part of routine nursing care that involves physical contact with a patient is examined so that subtle yet important ethical issues become salient.

Case Study

Bessie Watkins is a 5 ft, 10 in., 70-year-old retired school teacher who was admitted to the hospice care unit of a small community hospital. She was diagnosed with metastatic cancer that had spread from her left breast to her spine and ribs. Single and living in her own home with her only sister, she was admitted to the hospital because she had become too weak to walk and could barely feed herself. Upon the advice of her personal physician, Miss Watkins had decided not to undergo chemotherapy. Her admission orders noted that she was in the terminal stages of cancer and was to be kept comfortable with narcotic medication per continuous IV infusion.

Miss Watkins had many friends on the unit. Staff and visitors delighted in her bright wit, charm, sparkling eyes, and stories. But as the cancer spread throughout her body, she would cry and beg the staff not to move her by turning her. Because she was tall and thin, her bony prominences became more pronounced as she became sicker. A special mattress was ordered to help prevent breakdown of her skin, but the staff still needed to turn her several times a day to prevent pressure ulcers and to change the bed linens. When they did, Miss Watkins cried out from the pain so much that the staff wondered if they were really helping this patient by their nursing interventions.

Finally, the staff met to decide what they should do. Mrs. Twomey, the head nurse for 4 years, insisted that Miss Watkins be turned at least every 2–3 hours for linen changes and for observation of her skin. After all, she pointed out, that was routine and minimal nursing care for all bed-ridden patients, and this was the standard of the unit. Any skin breakdown and its necessary treatment would be a very serious problem for Miss Watkins in her already severely compromised condition. Mrs. Hanks, a nurse's aide on the unit for almost 15 years and a long-time acquaintance of Miss Watkins, said that she could not stand to see this patient cry every time she was turned. She said that she would prefer that Miss Watkins's sedation be increased to reduce her pain and facilitate linen changes. Miss Benson, a recent graduate, voiced her opinion that the patient should have some say regarding her care. After all, she had terminal cancer, and not turning her would hardly make a difference in the overall outcome of her illness. Mrs. Culver, the evening nurse, thought that her physician ought to be the one to decide how often Miss Watkins should be turned. Then, the nurses would not have to make a decision and could just follow his orders. The rest of the nurses strongly objected to this suggestion. Turning a patient, changing linen, and observing for skin breakdown are nursing measures, they argued, and they should decide together the appropriate nursing interventions for this patient. Could everyone be comfortable not turning Miss Watkins unless it was absolutely necessary? How should they decide? (Fry, Veatch, & Taylor, 2011, pp. 91–92)

Discussion

The question that closes this case study is not "*What* should they decide?" but rather "*How* should they decide?" By starting with a "how" question, the nursing care team has already made an important decision: They have decided that Miss Watkins' care is a communal decision that involves all members of the nursing team. The team members recognize their mutuality in caring for Miss Watkins, so the decision is collaborative, involving everyone who provides direct care to the patient. By so doing, care-based ethics is evident in the way the issue is handled. Additionally, another question is posed in the case study that focuses on the relationships that are an integral part of this patient's care: "Could everyone be comfortable . . . ?" directs attention to what it means to live with a moral decision and the recognition that decisions have far-reaching effects on those concerned. The decision of whether or not to turn Miss Watkins has ethical implications because it has a direct impact on human well-being, there does not appear to be one clearly correct course of action, and informed and well-intentioned individuals can disagree about which course of action is correct. When reviewing a case, sometimes the tendency is to find holes in the clinical problem so that the ethical issue disappears. In this case, some might argue that the newest bed and mattress system to prevent pressure ulcers could eliminate the problem of turning. That may be true, but the problem of keeping Miss Watkins clean and dry and the pain that results from those actions would remain, as would the larger issue of the appropriate trade-offs between pain and comfort in the case of a dying patient.

In the case of Miss Watkins, one could ask what the traditional ethical principles have to offer. If the light shines on the principle of respect for autonomy, there are more questions than answers. At one point, Miss Watkins appeared to have been competent because the case described "her bright wit, charm, sparkling eyes, and stories." When she was able to communicate, did anyone involve her in thinking about advance planning for her hospice care? Toward the end of the case, it seems that Miss Watkins is no longer capable of participating in her care and weighing the benefits or harms of turning her in bed as one of many decisions she might be asked to make. At this point, there is temptation to be judgmental about the evident lack of planning on the part of the staff involved in Miss Watkins' care, but placing blame does little to remedy the present problem. However, this experience with Miss Watkins might encourage the nursing staff involved to think differently about how they interact with future patients and when to address the subject of end-of-life care.

The principles of avoiding harm and doing good are also at work in this case as the individuals discuss minimal and routine care and standards. Generally speaking, maintaining skin integrity is a sign of good nursing care. Somehow in Miss Watkins' case, the routine good of turning a patient and changing soiled linens has become an instrument of pain with questionable outcomes. Members of the nursing team expressed their own pain that resulted from hearing Miss Watkins cry out, but all healthcare workers know that some pain is to be expected when delivering treatment. What makes Miss Watkins' cries intolerable for the team members? Indirect references to fidelity to the patient are most clearly highlighted by the nurse's aide, Mrs. Hanks, who has known the patient for a long time. Does the length of her relationship to Miss Watkins lend more weight to her comments about what should happen? Fidelity also plays a part in admission to a hospice care unit that promises certain assurances about end-of-life care. Hospice care, whether provided in someone's home, a skilled nursing facility, or a hospital unit, "embraces a philosophy of caring, combined with the best medical knowledge and clinical skills to provide care that is both compassionate and competent. In selecting hospice care, a dying person chooses health care that focuses on comfort and function rather than on cure or prolongation of life" (Lynn, Koshuta, & Schmitz, 1995, p. 1157). Miss Watkins chose hospice care on the recommendation of her physician. Choosing hospice means that Miss Watkins valued comfort rather than cure or prolongation of life. She should be able to rely on the implicit promises of a hospice program to deliver care directed to comfort. The final core principle, justice, does not seem to play a major role in helping analyze the case unless there is a sense that the team is somehow discriminating against Miss Watkins. If any unfairness exists in the case, it would seem to be toward a positive inclination to do right by this patient who "had many friends." One then sees how justice could play a significant role in the treatment of a patient who did not hold such esteem in the nursing team's collective heart.

Other factors certainly are involved in the cases that do not fit neatly into the principlist approach. For example, the members of the nursing team represent various positions and assigned status. Cohen and Erickson (2006) reflected on how different values and principles can move the characterization of the problem in a specific direction: "How an individual nurse perceives and reacts to a patient care situation is a highly individualized process that depends on the individual's unique set of beliefs and values. What one nurse sees as an ethical conflict may not be seen as troubling by another nurse who is guided by a different set of principles and priorities" (p. 777). Additionally, the experience of the nurse will reframe the problem, as can be seen with the new nurse, Miss Benson, who emphasized the patient's role in decision making, as compared to the seasoned head nurse, Mrs. Twomey, who appeared to value following a specific standard of care to avoid known harms (e.g., skin breakdown) regardless of the short-term pain to the patient. Miss Benson also argued that "not turning her would hardly make a difference," which gives insight into her assumption about whether others would share her view of the benefits and harms in the case.

Several tenets of care-based ethics resonated in the comments of the members of the nursing team. They are concerned about Miss Watkins as a person they know and care about. As a retired school teacher who possibly spent much of her life in the small community in which she is now hospitalized, Miss Watkins' connections to the nursing staff could be much more diverse than her present role as a patient. The case noted that Miss Watkins lived in her own home with her only sister, but there are no further references to this sister. It is unknown whether Miss Watkins and her sister were close or fought every day they lived together, nor if the sister was younger or older, sick or well, capacitated or incapacitated. It is only known that she is family. The sister may or may not be willing or able to participate in making decisions for her sister. One can assume that separation from her family and home is a drastic change in Miss Watkins' life, as she did her best to stay at home as long as she could. Involving the sister in a way that makes sense for both of them would seem to be an important connection to restore or at least explore. As Nelson and Nelson (1995) noted,

> In the midst of all the strangeness of illness or injury, alienated from ourselves and from the ongoing ordinariness of things, we can turn to our families for orientation to our new reality. The family's mechanisms for maintaining selves are never so useful as here, when we first begin to gauge the effect of bodily catastrophe on who we are. (p. 46)

The presence of Miss Watkins' sister will not necessarily solve the problem of whether or not to turn her as she lies dying, but it could make a dramatic difference in the quality of her dying. In addition to familial relationships, the relationships of the nursing staff to the patient and to each other are important. They are "standing" with Miss Watkins during this difficult time in her life, and they are working together to discuss how to make their actions "right." Mrs. Hanks even uses the metaphor of standing when she relates that she "could not stand to see this patient cry." Mrs. Hanks offered a sort of compromise resolution to the problem by suggesting increased sedation so that Miss Watkins would not be in pain when they turned her. This resolution takes care of the problem of pain and conforms to the standard nursing intervention for a bedridden patient, thereby fulfilling both moral obligations. Miss Benson would likely not share this view as she has already determined that turning is not providing enough benefit to outweigh the pain and thus is not a required intervention in this case.

Other questions remain that require careful balancing of principles as well as other ethical considerations that go beyond what principlism has to offer the individuals involved in Miss Watkins' care. The broader guiding principles that follow in the next section present some possibilities of looking beyond what should be done to the deeper meanings of actions.

A Broader Notion of Principles of Ethics

The following is an overview of five ethical considerations that have relevance in analyzing ethical issues in clinical practice. These considerations bridge a variety of perspectives and do not fit neatly into any particular category or approach to ethics. The first broad principle again involves reflection on benefits and harms but with additional parameters.

Proportionality in Clinical Decisions

When considering benefits and harms in the care of patients, it may be helpful to draw on the basic method of the Catholic tradition for resolving cases with complicated weighing of benefits and harms. Patients are at the center of this ethical focus that has gained traction in the secular world of healthcare ethics as well. Part Five of the *Ethical and Religious Directives for Catholic Health Care Services* states, "A person may forgo extraordinary or disproportionate means of preserving life. Disproportionate means are those that in the patient's judgment do not offer a reasonable hope of benefit or entail an excessive burden, or impose excessive expense on the family or the community" (United States Conference of Catholic Bishops, 2009, p. 31). The criterion of proportionality introduces the importance of intentionality when considering moral actions in addition to determining good and bad outcomes, some of which are intended whereas others are not. Proportionality argues that any evil caused by one's actions first must not be intentional, and second, must be counterbalanced by a proportionate good. Generally speaking, turning patients who are bedridden to avoid the harm of pressure ulcers is good; however, in the case of Miss Watkins, there is a predictable harm or evil—in this case, pain—that results from turning her that is not intentional yet happens nonetheless. Is this unintentional pain counterbalanced by the good that turning accomplishes? It is important to step back from the specifics of the case and think about the benefits and harms from the perspective of achieving treatment goals for all patients.

First, there is the presumption that the value and dignity of every patient demand treatment that is based on broad goals of health care that include cure (when possible), stabilization, restoration of bodily functions or mental capacity, and comfort. The treatment choice should always be based on the patient's best interest. Evidence of lack of proportionate benefit includes (1) the treatment would be futile, i.e., the patient would die regardless of the treatment, and the treatment merely serves to prolong the dying process, (2) "the potential for human relationship is non-existent or would be utterly submerged in intractable pain and/or the mere struggle to survive," or (3) when curative care is not possible, comforting and supportive care should become the goal (Glaser, 1985, pp. 89–90). One could argue that admission to hospice care by default determines certain types of care as inappropriate. There could also be strong arguments that turning is a futile treatment in the case of a dying patient. The assumption is that turning prevents pressure ulcers in dying patients, but is that assumption true? The nurses in Miss Watkins' case are not the only ones to ask questions about preventing and treating pressure ulcers in dying patients. If the nurses were to examine the literature on this topic, they would find a great deal of controversy. First, it appears that there are differences in the type of care provided depending on whether the goal is to prevent skin breakdown or to heal existing wounds. Also, a great deal of the effectiveness of nursing interventions depends on how close to death a patient is as well as other physiologic factors. As Hughes, Bakos, O'Mara, and Kovner (2005) noted, best practices for wound treatment in dying patients is a largely unexplored and complex topic.

Although there is not complete agreement, some research indicates that it is not possible to prevent pressure ulcers even with the most aggressive preventive care. Even if regular turning and skin care could indeed prevent skin breakdown, Miss Watkins and perhaps members of the nursing team might not agree with that goal of care. Comfort and support could take priority. A qualitative study of hospice directors and direct-care nurses regarding pressure ulcer treatment and prevention found that other goals may be more important to patients: "Comfort may supersede prevention and wound care when patients are actively dying or have conditions causing them to have a single position of comfort" (Eisenberger & Zeleznik, 2003, p. 19). The best care for Miss Watkins could be to leave her in a comfortable position and only provide care that keeps her clean and warm, with appropriate pain management when it is necessary to move her. Such a plan would be in line with the following admonition from ONS.

> Dying people are cared for by compassionate, sensitive, and knowledgeable professionals who attempt to identify, understand, and meet their individual needs, particularly in the case of fear or a sense of hopelessness or loss of control. Alleviation of pain and other serious symptoms must be a key priority in providing quality palliative care. (ONS, 2010, p. 249)

Distinguishing Between Pain and Suffering

Beyond balancing adequate pain relief, comfort, and possibly consciousness, the clinical case calls for the distinction between pain and suffering. Nurses are particularly situated in health care to be present to suffering. Even with careful and individualized assessment, planning, and treatment for pain in a dying patient, suffering can and often does occur. In Miss Watkins' case, she could not speak with words but communicated powerfully through her cries of pain. Her suffering also affected those who cared for her. As Fowler (2008) noted, "Suffering can make us acutely aware of our mortality and impotence, dashing our illusions of control and power, and yet it can move us to develop in new ways, ways that joy does not" (p. 274). The members of the nursing team were used to doing things to and for patients, but when a patient is dying, there is generally less to do regarding treatments and medications. When there is less rushing about and "doing," nurses have to face what is happening. They may lose the comfort of being in action and the sense of control it gives. What is required, then, is to be present to suffering. Fowler explained, "This presence is a presence in vulnerability—the vulnerability of the shared human condition—that, while it still retains identity boundaries, is open to an ontological change in both persons by virtue of human connectedness" (p. 276). The nursing team caring for Miss Watkins must accept not only her death but also their own vulnerability and limitations while carrying on with other patients and families. Dealing with suffering on the part of patients and health professionals has clear ethical implications and is an often-neglected yet important component of ethical analysis.

Disclosure, Informed Consent, and Shared Decision Making

The time for discussion about treatment options and planning for care has passed for Miss Watkins. When she was able to participate, critical conversations did not seem to take place, which might have been helpful at this juncture in making treatment decisions that were in accordance with her wishes and goals. However, in most cases, the foundational principles of disclosing understandable information and engaging the patient and family in decision making are critical. As noted by Fletcher and Spencer (2005),

> Healthcare, particularly when alternative treatments are possible, inevitably involves issues of values, which do not lie within the domain of medical knowledge. How can clinicians determine, in all cases, what is in the best interest of patients without consulting patients and adequately disclosing what they need to know to make decisions? (p. 13)

Miss Benson noted this important aspect of the basic underlying ethical components of respect for autonomy in her comments. If possible, patients should be involved in discussions and decision making, and decisions should be revisited if the situation changes. Additionally, many small but important treatment questions should be addressed even if the established goal is comfort. Then, with this foundation of shared decision making, even when a patient can no longer participate in decisions, the treatment team has insight into what the patient would want. As Cain and Hammes (1994) stated, "Information that can be considered by patients, families and their physicians at a time when impending crisis management is not looming large represents a greater respect for encouraging accurate expressions of wishes and values" (p. 162).

Fulfilling Professional Responsibilities and Integrity

The process of restoring health, wholeness, or healing depends on the trust of patients and their families and the trustworthiness of health professionals. Clinicians owe patients not only their competency but also their dedication to clear and sustained communication. Additionally, health professionals owe patients a caring presence. All of this sounds very simple, yet in practice it can be very difficult for health professionals to care for someone who has a life-limiting illness or who is suffering. Not only is it important to "do" the right thing, but the manner in which a health professional interacts with a patient and family is equally important.

There is specific expression of concern in the clinical case about the integrity of those involved in Miss Watkins' care when they ask, "Could everyone be comfortable . . . ?" What sort of treatment plan and course of care can everyone involved in Miss Watkins' care live with in the immediate future and after her death? Although not the case here, sometimes clinicians are asked to provide treatment that is in opposition to their consciences. Patients have the right to refuse treatments, but they do not have the right to request treatments that are inappropriate or that would undermine the health professional's integrity. ANA's *Code of Ethics for Nurses* supports this obligation in Provision 5, which states, "The nurse owes the same duties to self as to others, including the responsibility to promote health and safety, preserve wholeness of character and integrity, maintain competence, and continue personal and professional growth" (ANA, 2015, p. 19). The idea of integrity bridges the personal and professional elements of identity. Integrity is informed by experiences that reshape what it means to be a good health professional.

Considerations of Power

The patient and family are always in a position of diminished authority because of illness, injury, less education, and position within the healthcare system. Sharing understandable information and allowing adequate time and dialogue for understanding are ways to balance power differentials. Another way to equalize power is to consider the specific implications of the patient and his or her family so that care is personalized. This case involves specific nursing interventions unlike other interventions that belong to other disciplines or are shared, such as end-of-life treatment decisions that include do-not-resuscitate orders or withholding or withdrawing artificial nutrition and hydration. When Mrs. Culver suggested shifting responsibility to the physician for the decision so they could "just follow orders," there was immediate pushback by her peers. The specific intervention is under the nurses' purview. Therefore, it was up to "them" to decide, and they resisted relinquishing their power to a higher authority. If nurses claim power, then they need to accept the responsibility that goes with it, including being competent in all aspects of the literature on skin care and dying patients as well as the ethical basis for decisions to withhold standard therapy.

Other members of the healthcare team are in positions of diminished authority, such as nursing assistants and aides. Such individuals also bear witness to patients' suffering and may be in a unique position to notify professionals higher up on the organizational ladder about their concerns. In fact, nursing assistants often feel morally responsible to call attention to issues because of the intimate care they provide and the relationships that are established from such involvement with patients

(McClement, Lobchuk, Chochinov, & Dean, 2010; McClement, Wowchuk, & Klaasen, 2009). In Miss Watkins' case, the nurse's aide, Mrs. Hanks, not only is part of the discussion but feels empowered enough in the group to speak up and offer a possible resolution to the conflicts in the patient's care. By minimizing power differentials, it becomes possible to hear and respect every voice, which adds to the probability of reaching a sound decision that the team can accept.

Conclusion

Ethical principles can be a source of guidance for oncology nurses as they steer a course through complicated clinical dilemmas. However, the moral life is more than making discrete decisions but encompasses how nurses live and think about these important ethical matters. To avoid a too-narrow view of ethical discernment, broader concepts of principles, such as proportionality, considerations of power, and facilitating shared decision making, are necessary to consider the variety of issues at play. The question of how to do good for a patient in oncology nursing leads to other more profound questions that take into account the wider ethical considerations of caring for others within a complex healthcare delivery system and the broader society in which it exists.

References

American Nurses Association. (2013). Position statement on euthanasia, assisted suicide, and aid in dying. Retrieved from http://www.nursingworld.org/MainMenuCategories/EthicsStandards/Ethics-Position-Statements/Euthanasia-Assisted-Suicide-and-Aid-in-Dying.pdf

American Nurses Association. (2015). Code of ethics for nurses with interpretive statements. Retrieved from http://www.nursingworld.org/MainMenuCategories/EthicsStandards/CodeofEthicsforNurses

Arras, J.D. (1994). Principles and particularity: The role of cases in bioethics. Indiana Law Journal, 69, 983–1014.

Beauchamp, T.L., & Childress, J.F. (2012). Principles of biomedical ethics (7th ed.). New York, NY: Oxford University Press.

Blackhall, L.J., Frank, G., Murphy, S., & Michel, V. (2001). Bioethics in a different tongue: The case of truth-telling. Journal of Urban Health, 78, 59–71. doi:10.1093/jurban/78.1.59

Cain, J.M., & Hammes, B.J. (1994). Ethics and pain management: Respecting patient wishes. Journal of Pain and Symptom Management, 9, 160–165. doi:10.1016/0885-3924(94)90125-2

Childress, J.F. (1982). Who should decide? Paternalism in health care. New York, NY: Oxford University Press.

Clouser, K.D., & Gert, B. (1990). A critique of principlism. Journal of Medicine and Philosophy, 15, 219–236. doi:10.1093/jmp/15.2.219

Cohen, J.S., & Erickson, J.M. (2006). Ethical dilemmas and moral distress in oncology nursing practice. Clinical Journal of Oncology Nursing, 10, 775–780. doi:10.1188/06.CJON.775-780

Collopy, B.J. (1988). Autonomy in long term care: Some crucial distinctions. Gerontologist, 28(Suppl.), 10–17. doi:10.1093/geront/28.Suppl.10

Davis, A.J., Aroskar, M.A., Liaschenko, J., & Drought, T.S. (1997). Ethical dilemmas and nursing practice (4th ed.). Stamford, CT: Appleton and Lange.

Dougherty, C.J., Edwards, B.J., & Haddad, A.M. (1990). *Ethical dilemmas in perioperative nursing.* Denver, CO: Association of Operating Room Nurses.

Edelstein, L. (1987). The Hippocratic Oath: Text, translation and interpretation. In O. Temkin & C.L. Temkin (Eds.), *Ancient medicine: Selected papers of Ludwig Edelstein* (pp. 3–64). Baltimore, MD: Johns Hopkins Press.

Eisenberger, A., & Zeleznik, J. (2003). Pressure ulcer prevention and treatment in hospices: A qualitative analysis. *Journal of Palliative Care, 19,* 9–14.

Fletcher, J.C., & Spencer, E.M. (2005). Clinical ethics: History, content and resources. In J.C. Fletcher, E.M. Spencer, & P.A. Lombardo (Eds.), *Fletcher's introduction to clinical ethics* (pp. 3–18). Hagerstown, MD: University Publishing Group.

Fowler, M.D.M. (2008). Come; give me a taste of shalom. In W.E. Pinch & A.M. Haddad (Eds.), *Nursing and health care ethics: A legacy and a vision* (pp. 269–281). Silver Spring, MD: American Nurses Association.

Fry, S.T., Veatch, R.M., & Taylor, C. (2011). *Case studies in nursing ethics* (4th ed.). Burlington, MA: Jones & Bartlett Learning.

Fullam, L. (2006, December). Virtue ethics: An introduction. *Journal of Lutheran Ethics, 6*(12). Retrieved from http://downloads.elca.org/html/jle/www.elca.org/what-we-believe/social-issues/virtue-ethics-an-introduction.aspx.htm

Glaser, J. (1985). *Caring for the special child.* Kansas City, MO: Leaven Press.

Glaser, J. (1994). *Three realms of ethics.* Kansas City, MO: Sheed and Ward.

Hospice and Palliative Nurses Association. (2011). Role of the nurse when hastened death is requested [Position statement]. Retrieved from http://hpna.advancingexpertcare.org/wp-content/uploads/2015/08/Role-of-the-Nurse-When-Hastened-Death-is-Requested.pdf

Hughes, R.G., Bakos, A.D., O'Mara, A., & Kovner, C.T. (2005). Palliative wound care at the end of life. *Home Health Care Management and Practice, 17,* 196–202. doi:10.1177/1084822304271815

Jecker, N.S., & Reich, W.T. (1995). Contemporary ethics of care. In W.T. Reich (Ed.), *Encyclopedia of bioethics* (2nd ed., pp. 336–344). New York, NY: Macmillan.

Little, M.O. (1996). Why a feminist approach to bioethics? *Kennedy Institute of Ethics Journal, 6,* 1–18. doi:10.1353/ken.1996.0005

Lynn, J., Koshuta, M., & Schmitz, P. (1995). Hospice and end-of-life care. In W.T. Reich (Ed.), *Encyclopedia of bioethics* (2nd ed., pp. 1157–1159). New York, NY: Macmillan.

McClement, S., Lobchuk, M., Chochinov, H.M., & Dean, R. (2010). Broken covenant: Healthcare aides' "experience of the ethical" in caring for dying seniors in a personal care home. *Journal of Clinical Ethics, 21,* 201–211.

McClement, S., Wowchuk, S., & Klaasen, K. (2009). "Caring as if it were my family": Health care aides' perspectives about expert care of the dying resident in a personal care home. *Palliative and Supportive Care, 7,* 449–457. doi:10.1017/S1478951509990459

National Commission for the Protection of Human Subjects of Biomedical and Behavioral Research. (1979, April 18). *The Belmont Report: Ethical principles and guidelines for the protection of human subjects of research.* Retrieved from http://www.hhs.gov/ohrp/humansubjects/guidance/belmont.html

Nelson, H.L., & Nelson, J.L. (1995). *The patient in the family: An ethics of medicine and families.* New York, NY: Routledge.

Oncology Nursing Society. (2010). Nurses' responsibility to patients requesting assistance in hastening death [Position statement]. *Oncology Nursing Forum, 37,* 249–250.

Ramsey, P. (2002). *The patient as person: Explorations in medical ethics* (2nd ed.). New Haven, CT: Yale University Press.

Storch, J.L., Rodney, P., & Starzomski, R.C. (Eds.). (2004). *Toward a moral horizon: Nursing ethics for leadership and practice.* Toronto, Ontario, Canada: Pearson Prentice Hall.

United States Conference of Catholic Bishops. (2009). *Ethical and religious directives for Catholic health care services* (5th ed.). Retrieved from http://www.usccb.org/about/doctrine/ethical-and-religious-directives

Veatch, R.M. (1981). *A theory of medical ethics.* New York, NY: Basic Books.

Veatch, R.M., & Haddad, A. (2008). *Case studies in pharmacy ethics* (2nd ed.). New York, NY: Oxford University Press.

Veatch, R.M., Haddad, A.M., & English, D.C. (2010). *Case studies in biomedical ethics: Decision-making, principles, and cases.* New York, NY: Oxford University Press.

Viafora, C. (1999). Toward a methodology for the ethical analysis of clinical practice. *Medicine, Health Care and Philosophy, 2,* 283–297.

CHAPTER 2

Medical Research and Clinical Trials

Rose Ermete, RN, BSN, OCN®, CCRP

Introduction

Ethics in medical research involves moral principles that guide research practice (Hardicre, 2014). Virtually every aspect of a clinical trial, from inception through reporting of results, has ethical implications. Often, participants are patients undergoing treatment at the same time and by the same healthcare provider, and protecting their rights and well-being is paramount. The roles of researcher and clinician can sometimes be in conflict, and when attempting to answer a critical research question, scientists may have difficulty determining what is ethical. Throughout history, atrocities have occurred related to the lack of patient protections. Investigators in these studies may have justified their views on the basis that the work would yield results for the good of society and would otherwise be unprocurable with protections in place. This form of thought ignores patient autonomy, one of the basic tenets of research ethics. Laws and regulations have been established to protect patients' rights. Nurses must adhere to these regulations and ethical principles when involved in clinical trials to ensure the collection of quality data and protect the rights and well-being of patients (Oncology Nursing Society, 2010).

Historical Review of Ethical Principles in Research

The Nuremberg Code

Several documents exist that embody the ethics of clinical trials. The first of these documents is the Nuremberg Code (see Figure 2-1). The Nuremberg Code

Figure 2-1. The Nuremberg Code

1. The voluntary consent of the human subject is absolutely essential.
   - This means that the person involved should have legal capacity to give consent; should be so situated as to be able to exercise free power of choice, without the intervention of any element of force, fraud, deceit, duress, over-reaching, or other ulterior form of constraint or coercion; and should have sufficient knowledge and comprehension of the elements of the subject matter involved as to enable him to make an understanding and enlightened decision. This latter element requires that before the acceptance of an affirmative decision by the experimental subject there should be made known to him the nature, duration, and purpose of the experiment; the method and means by which it is to be conducted; all inconveniences and hazards reasonably to be expected; and the effects upon his health or person which may possibly come from his participation in the experiment.
   - The duty and responsibility for ascertaining the quality of the consent rests upon each individual who initiates, directs, or engages in the experiment. It is a personal duty and responsibility which may not be delegated to another with impunity.
2. The experiment should be such as to yield fruitful results for the good of society, unprocurable by other methods or means of study, and not random and unnecessary in nature.
3. The experiment should be so designed and based on the results of animal experimentation and a knowledge of the natural history of the disease or other problem under study that the anticipated results will justify the performance of the experiment.
4. The experiment should be so conducted as to avoid all unnecessary physical and mental suffering and injury.
5. No experiment should be conducted where there is an *a priori* reason to believe that death or disabling injury will occur; except, perhaps, in those experiments where the experimental physicians also serve as subjects.
6. The degree of risk to be taken should never exceed that determined by the humanitarian importance of the problem to be solved by the experiment.
7. Proper preparations should be made and adequate facilities provided to protect the experimental subject against even remote possibilities of injury, disability, or death.
8. The experiment should be conducted only by scientifically qualified persons. The highest degree of skill and care should be required through all stages of the experiment of those who conduct or engage in the experiment.
9. During the course of the experiment, the human subject should be at liberty to bring the experiment to an end if he has reached the physical or mental state where continuation of the experiment seems to him to be impossible.
10. During the course of the experiment, the scientist in charge must be prepared to terminate the experiment at any stage, if he has probably cause to believe, in the exercise of the good faith, superior skill, and careful judgment required of him, that a continuation of the experiment is likely to result in injury, disability, or death to the experimental subject.

Note. From *Trials of War Criminals Before the Nuernberg Military Tribunals Under Control Council Law No. 10* (Vol. 2, pp. 181–182), 1949. Retrieved from http://www.loc.gov/rr/frd/Military_Law/pdf/NT_war-criminals_Vol-II.pdf.

was established as a result of the International Military Tribunal at Nuremberg for war crimes resulting from murderous and torturous human experiments in Nazi concentration camps during World War II. During the war, camp physicians conducted many unethical experiments on human subjects without consent. In one example, wounds were inflicted on subjects and then infected with bacteria, wood shavings, and ground glass to mimic those found on the battlefield. Healthy subjects were also infected with various bacteria. During the tribunal, it was established that these subjects unwillingly participated under duress and coercion, suffering physical torture and sometimes dying from unbeneficial experiments. The tribunal found that the core offense was misconduct based on lack of voluntary consent. The Nuremberg Code was the first document to articulate ethical standards of behavior applicable to all people conducting research with human subjects (Nuremberg Code, 1949).

The Declaration of Helsinki

The Nuremberg Code was a precursor to the Universal Declaration of Human Rights, which was adopted by the United Nations in 1948. However, it would seem that this document was not thought to be necessary for American physicians. Bioethicist Jay Katz described the prevalent attitude at that time, stating, "It was a good code for barbarians, but an unnecessary code for ordinary physicians" (Parascandola, 2000, p. 39). In the aftermath of one of the most significant medical abuses, the thalidomide disaster, the 18th World Medical Association General Assembly of 1964 adopted a resolution on human experimentation, the Declaration of Helsinki. The document had its basis in the Nuremberg Code; however, it went a step further by addressing the need for a review by an ethics committee and by expanding on informed consent:

> In case of legal incompetence, informed consent should be obtained from the legal guardian in accordance with national legislation. Where physical or mental incapacity makes it impossible to obtain informed consent, or when the subject is a minor, permission from the responsible relative replaces that of the subject in accordance with national legislation. Whenever the minor child is in fact able to give a consent, the minor's consent must be obtained in addition to the consent of the minor's legal guardian. (World Medical Association, 1996)

The Nuremberg Code listed several principles to ensure the rights and protection of those participating in research. However, the determination of whether a study was ethical was left to the individual investigators. Investigators may have many competing interests (e.g., obtaining funding, enhancing a career, completing research in a timely fashion, maintaining financial interests with various companies) that could cloud their determination (Emanuel, Wendler, & Grady, 2000). The Declaration of Helsinki requires an independent review of a research study by an ethics committee before it can commence. This review helps minimize any potential conflicts of interest and provides further protection from exploitation of research subjects.

Unlike the Nuremberg Code, the Declaration of Helsinki is a living document. It is reviewed and revised at regular intervals as cultures and values change over time. Since its inception in 1964, it has been revised nine times, most recently in October 2013, to address new concerns as they arise. The original document provided 12 basic principles, an explanation of medical research combined with professional care, and an explanation of nontherapeutic biomedical research involving human subjects. The current document has been expanded and now covers 37 principles (World Medical Association, 2013).

Research in the United States

The recommendations of the Declaration of Helsinki were not made law or proposed in any regulations at the time of the document's creation. However, in 1966, grant recipients within the U.S. Public Health Service were required to provide documentation of compliance with these ethical standards prior to trial initiation and the award of funds (Saunders, 1995). It took the exposure of several unethical practices in human research experiments in the United States to prompt Congress to create laws to ensure the safety of participants and the validity of research studies.

In 1966, Henry Beecher published an article in the *New England Journal of Medicine* that described several unethical research projects conducted at prestigious institutions. Generally, these studies were conducted to improve the understanding of disease, yet they had no clinical benefit to the subjects involved.

One of these studies was conducted at Willowbrook State School, a former institution on New York City's Staten Island for children with learning disabilities. The school was closed to new students because of overcrowding. However, prospective students were admitted if their parent agreed to let them participate in the study. Investigators wanted to determine the period of infectivity of hepatitis. The children were initially fed extracts of feces from known infected children and later were given an intramuscular injection with the virus (Hardicre, 2014; Hornblum, Newman, & Dober, 2013). These children were unnecessarily exposed to hepatitis for the benefit of understanding the disease and developing a vaccine (Parascandola, 2000).

Another study discussed by Beecher was conducted at the Jewish Chronic Disease Hospital in Brooklyn, New York. The purpose of this study was to understand the immune response of cancer. Liver cancer cells were injected into senile older adult patients (McNeilly, 2011). They were not told they were injected with cancer cells; instead, they were informed they were receiving "some cells." There was also no documentation of consent (Beecher, 1966). Beecher noted, "It is evident that in many of the examples presented, the investigators have risked the health or the life of their subjects" (p. 1356).

Another highly unethical and widely publicized study occurred in Tuskegee, Alabama, in 1932 (Hardicre, 2014; McNeilly, 2011; Parascandola, 2000). This study by the U.S. Public Health Service involved observing the course of syphilis in African American men, all of whom were poor and uneducated. The participants were told they had "bad blood," not that they had syphilis. They were given hot meals, medical insurance for simple treatments, and free burial insurance. The participants thought they were receiving treatment; however, they only received aspirin, placebos, or vitamin tablets (Hardicre, 2014; Parascandola, 2000). In 1947, penicillin became available and was the drug of choice for the treatment of syphilis. The participants in this study were not informed of this treatment option (McNeilly, 2011). This experiment continued until 1972, when public outcry forced Congress to act.

The Belmont Report

In 1974, Congress passed the National Research Act. This created the National Commission for the Protection of Human Subjects of Biomedical and Behavioral Research. The commission's charge was to identify basic ethical principles when conducting research on human subjects and to develop guidelines to ensure compliance with those principles. The document they developed is known as the Belmont Report, released on April 18, 1979, and is one of the leading documents in clinical research ethics (National Commission for the Protection of Human Subjects of Biomedical and Behavioral Research, 1979). It continues to serve as the basic ethical guideline and foundation for the regulations that govern clinical trials.

The Belmont Report is based on three ethical principles: respect for persons, beneficence, and justice. Respect for persons values both autonomy and protection of those with diminished autonomy (McNeilly, 2011). Autonomy refers to the ability of an individual to independently make a decision. Autonomy can be disrespected by denying individuals the freedom to act on their own interpretations or by withholding necessary information from individuals when there is no reason to do so (National Commission for the Protection of Human Subjects of Biomedical and Behavioral Research, 1979). To remain compliant with this principle, the study staff need to obtain voluntary informed consent from subjects prior to conducting any study procedure. In some cases, individuals may not be able to give their informed consent. In these cases, it is crucial to provide extra protection and obtain informed consent from a legally authorized representative (Sims, 2010).

The second principle is that of beneficence, encompassing two additional values: to do no harm and to maximize possible benefits and minimize possible harms (National Commission for the Protection of Human Subjects of Biomedical and Behavioral Research, 1979). At times, it is necessary to expose a subject to risks in order to achieve a benefit. When participants are exposed to risks, the benefits must outweigh those risks. The risk-benefit ratio needs to be considered by the investigator, as well as the independent ethics committee or institutional review board (IRB), when designing a study.

Justice is the third principle of the Belmont Report, referring to the equal distribution of research burdens and benefits (McNeilly, 2011). Acceptance or rejection of a study participant cannot be based on factors unrelated to the research. It is unethical for one group to endure the burdens and risks while another group experiences the benefits. During the 19th and early 20th centuries, the poor and the wards of the state bore the burdens of research, while the benefits flowed primarily to private patients (National Commission for the Protection of Human Subjects of Biomedical and Behavioral Research, 1979). From the several studies discussed previously, one can see that subject selection was frequently made for reasons unrelated to the study, including ease of availability or manipulability (i.e., people in a compromised state). Justice also demands that advantages are provided not only to those who can afford them and that such research should not unduly involve people from groups unlikely to benefit from the application of the research findings (National Commission for the Protection of Human Subjects of Biomedical and Behavioral Research, 1979).

The Belmont Report is grounded in the same principles cited in the Nuremberg Code and the Declaration of Helsinki. It provides guiding principles that help resolve ethical problems related to clinical research (Liu & Davis, 2010). This document was printed in the *Federal Register* in April 1979. The federal regulations that followed were based on the Belmont Report and other works of the commission. The regulations provide a legal framework that honors ethical principles, giving investigators a legal obligation to conduct ethical research (21 C.F.R. pt. 50, 2014; 21 C.F.R. pt. 56, 2014). These regulations mandated informed consent, equitable selection of subjects, and review by an impartial group of people with the goal of protecting those who take part in the study. This group can be known as an ethics committee, ethics review board, or IRB. Unethical research practices under the regulations that establish and govern the IRB could result in fines, disbarment, or even imprisonment.

The historical review of the three documents discussed provides an overview of the development of research ethics. The Nuremberg Code, the Declaration of Helsinki, and the Belmont Report provide the foundation for ethical practices and laws and regulations in the conduct of human research. Nurses and other healthcare professionals should have a thorough understanding of these principles to ensure the protection of the rights and well-being of patients involved in research.

Ethical Implications in Clinical Trials

Several steps in the research process require application of ethical principles. These steps will be discussed, as well as where to find information about each topic in the study documents. Oncology nurses also should consider the research staff, coordinators, and IRB as resources to better understand the study or to discuss concerns.

Study Design

The foundation of any ethical clinical trial is a well-designed study. To ensure patient protection and nonexploitation, researchers and study staff need to consider numerous factors when developing a clinical trial. In addition, a poorly designed trial will not provide an answer to the research question, making it very unlikely that society will benefit (Sachs, 2009). This not only wastes limited resources, but more importantly, it unnecessarily exposes the participants to risks. If the study cannot generate valid scientific knowledge, it is unethical (Emanuel et al., 2000).

A scientifically sound study should ensure that clinical equipoise exists. This means that no evidence exists that supports a difference between the interventions, or that there is uncertainty within the scientific community that a difference exists (Ubel & Silbergleit, 2011). Therefore, the research question is based on a true null hypothesis (Schlichting, 2010). In a randomized clinical trial, a null hypothesis is usually the supposition that sample observations result purely from chance. A trial tries to disprove the null, with the belief that the new intervention has an effect that is greater than chance. Further, if consensus is that the proposed intervention is not at least comparable to the current standard of care, it would be unethical to offer participation to patients, as they may receive substandard care (Chambers, 2011). *Standard of care* in research refers to care that should be provided based on established, effective, and proven methods for a given disease or healthcare problem (van der Graaf & van Delden, 2009). Randomizing patients to a substandard therapy goes against the ethical principle of beneficence and could be considered exploitation. The information in the background section of the protocol is a good resource to review in assessing whether clinical equipoise exists. This protocol section discusses the scientific rationale for the study, including prior studies and whether there is consensus.

The statistical section of the protocol should also be reviewed. A study should have sufficient power to determine if the results will be valid and clinically useful, meaning it can detect clinically significant differences. The definition of power, as noted by Cadeddu et al. (2008), is the ability of a study to detect an effect or association if one really exists in a wider population.

When a study has sufficient power, type I and II errors are less likely to occur (Sargent, 2014). *Type I errors* refer to a false positive, which is the chance that the study concludes there is a difference when there is no difference. *Type II errors* refer to a false negative, which is the failure to detect a minimum clinically important difference when there is one. Type I errors are set at 0.05. This is the significance level (p value). Type II errors are set at 0.2, usually reported as a percentage. This refers to the chance of detecting a difference at 80%, with a 20% chance of missing the difference (Sargent, 2014).

For a study to have greater power, a large sample size is needed. However, the sample size also depends on the size of the effect. *Effect size* refers to the minimum difference between two or more groups that would result in a change in patient management (Cadeddu et al., 2008), or how large a difference between the two means would be of scientific or clinical interest. If the effect size is small, a larger sample size is required; if the effect size is large, a smaller sample size is needed. As explained by Cohen (1988), the values of 0.2, 0.4, or 0.8 should be considered small, medium, and large effect sizes, respectively. The purpose of reviewing the statistical section of the study is to ensure that the study is designed to detect whether there is a difference between the dissimilar interventions. Again, it would be unethical to expose subjects to risk or inconvenience if this cannot be determined and no conclusions can be made.

Two other factors to consider when evaluating a study are fair subject selection and a favorable risk-benefit ratio. If both of these exist, the chance of exploitation of subjects is minimized. The fairness of subject selection goes hand in hand with the justice principle of the Belmont Report. The study should state how subjects will be selected, including whether certain populations are excluded and where and how subjects will be recruited. If a certain population is excluded, a scientific reason should be given. The population that bears the risks and burdens of the research should also enjoy its benefits, just as those who may benefit should also share some of the risks and burdens (Emanuel et al., 2000).

Risk-benefit ratio refers to the comparison of the amount of risk versus the amount of benefit. Beneficence is the foundation of the risk-benefit ratio. Risks should always be minimized, and benefits enhanced (National Commission for the Protection of Human Subjects of Biomedical and Behavioral Research, 1979). Many times in oncologic clinical trials, significant risk is associated with the study intervention. For many patients, particularly those with no treatment options, the possibility that the study may offer any benefit—no matter how small—outweighs the risks of study participation. This is especially true of the first three phases of a clinical trial (particularly phase I), where the focus is on safety and effectiveness.

Phase I studies involve a small number of patients. Researchers are trying to determine the safe dosage range and identify the side effects of a new drug or treatment. The patient's benefit is not the focus. In phase II, the new drug or treatment is given to a larger group of people to see if it is effective and to further evaluate its safety. In phase III trials, the drug or treatment is given to a much larger group of people to confirm its effectiveness, monitor side effects, compare it to commonly used treatments, and collect information that will allow the drug or treatment to be used safely (National Cancer Institute [NCI], 2014).

None of these phases are without risks. One way of minimizing the risks to participants is to review the adverse events of the treatment being offered. This information is located in the drug section of the protocol. In many cases, certain conditions may be exacerbated by the administration of a study agent. Participants with those conditions should be excluded from the study, as their risk would be considerably higher. Certain medicines also may be contraindicated for concurrent use with the study agent. If participants cannot stop the contraindicated medicine safely, they should be excluded as well. Other protocol sections to review include treatment modification and early stopping rules. Most studies require an intervention to be held or stopped if certain toxicities occur. This is another built-in safety protection for patients, as some risks may not be known.

A last thing to mention related to benefits is that paying participants and providing routine healthcare services are not considered benefits. Providing money, other than nominal amounts for transportation or similar inconveniences, can be viewed as coercive. Moreover, money is not seen as a health benefit (Sachs, 2009).

Informed Consent

Informed consent is the foundation for patient protection and an essential element of ethical research. It is not the paper that is being presented and signed, nor the initial discussion, but rather an ongoing process throughout the conduct of the trial. Chambers (2011) described the process as "the autonomous choice among alternative courses of action under conditions of risk" (p. 138). As discussed previously, autonomy demonstrates respect for the individual. To respect a person is to value his or her decision and to allow a change of mind as new information becomes available. Parker (2010) discussed relevant moral standards that guide behavior and actions. These are largely based on the primacy principle, which is the concept that the human individual is the criterion of value in human life. In clinical trials, this principle guides behaviors and actions. To abide by this principle is to attribute value to moral standards. Moral standards are a set of restraints on action in the care of individuals, such as do not take advantage of and do not harm people (Parker, 2010). In the United States, these moral standards for informed consent have been codified in 21 C.F.R. § 50.20 (see Figure 2-2). For informed consent to be truly voluntary and for patients to make an informed decision, all information about the research must be shared with potential participants. Parker (2010) argued that without fully informed consent, there is no clear difference between modern-day research subjects and the victims of Nazi experimentation. If further information is discovered that would change the rational decision the subject has committed to, it must be shared. Otherwise, it would not be ethical to obtain the consent (Chambers, 2011).

The *Code of Federal Regulations* (21 C.F.R. § 50.25) lists eight elements to be communicated to each potential subject (see Figure 2-3). The subject must be informed that this is a research study; it cannot be called a program or "new" treatment. The individual needs to know it is experimental. Risks cannot be minimized; all risks must be discussed. In some studies, there may be no direct benefit to the patient. In these cases, this must be explained. Some patients may consider altruism as a benefit, where research participants are motivated by a concern for the good of others when there may be no benefit to themselves (Jansen, 2009). Payment for participation is not considered a benefit and should not be described as such (Sachs,

---

Figure 2-2. General Requirements for Informed Consent

Except as provided in 50.23 and 50.24, no investigator may involve a human being as a subject in research covered by these regulations unless the investigator has obtained the legally effective informed consent of the subject or the subject's legally authorized representative. An investigator shall seek such consent only under circumstances that provide the prospective subject or the representative sufficient opportunity to consider whether or not to participate and that minimize the possibility of coercion or undue influence. The information that is given to the subject or the representative shall be in language understandable to the subject or the representative. No informed consent, whether oral or written, may include any exculpatory language through which the subject or the representative is made to waive or appear to waive any of the subject's legal rights, or releases or appears to release the investigator, the sponsor, the institution, or its agents from liability for negligence.

Note. From 21 C.F.R. § 50.20 (2014). Retrieved from http://www.accessdata.fda.gov/scripts/cdrh/ cfdocs/cfCFR/CFRSearch.cfm?CFRPart=50&showFR=1.

2009). Alternatives to the research study may include the option of no treatment at all. The current known outcomes of alternatives can be discussed. Health Insurance Portability and Accountability Act (HIPAA) consent is required to inform potential subjects about confidentiality protections. This can be part of the main consent document or a separate form. The informed consent document must state that the subject may discontinue participation at any time (21 C.F.R. § 50.25). Section 50.25 lists six additional elements that must be disclosed to the patient if applicable (see Figure 2-3). In addition, all NCI Cancer Therapy Evaluation Program (CTEP)-sponsored studies are required to provide notice that the description of the trial is available online at www.clinicaltrials.gov (NCI CTEP, 2013).

Ensuring the protection of vulnerable subjects is also paramount. This may include children, prisoners, pregnant women, physically or mentally disabled people, or people who are economically or educationally disadvantaged. As 21 C.F.R. § 56.111 explains, these people are likely to be vulnerable to coercion or undue influence. In these cases, the study must include additional safeguards to protect the rights and welfare of these subjects. For example, Meneguin and Ayres (2014) discussed several factors related to socioeconomic conditions that limit a person's understanding of the consent, such as anxiety and cultural and emotional barriers. These people may volunteer because of their difficulties accessing healthcare services in general. They may agree to participate because they believe that the clinical trial can offer some benefit. This is considered a therapeutic misconception, as the study may not offer a direct benefit to current participants. Participants need to understand that the research intervention may or may not provide benefit and that care is being partially directed by a protocol and not necessarily as preferred by the treating clinician (Schlichting, 2010). If study subjects are illiterate, they may not understand the informed consent process. The *Code of Federal Regulations* requires that information be offered in language understandable to the subject (21 C.F.R. § 50.20). This becomes a challenge with the increasing complexity of protocols and in individuals who have cognitive impairment or low to moderate health literacy.

Investigative sites, in collaboration with IRBs, should consider diverse methods to ensure understanding in these circumstances. Palmer (2013) discussed several suggestions to increase study subjects' understanding, including a teach-back

---

Figure 2-3. Basic Elements of Informed Consent

1. A statement that the study involves research, an explanation of the purposes of the research and the expected duration of the subject's participation, a description of the procedures to be followed, and identification of any procedures which are experimental.
2. A description of any reasonably foreseeable risks or discomforts to the subject.
3. A description of any benefits to the subject or to others which may reasonably be expected from the research.
4. A discloser of appropriate alternative procedures or courses of treatment.
5. A statement describing the extent, if any, to which confidentiality of records identifying the subject will be maintained and that notes the possibility that the Food and Drug Administration may inspect the records.
6. For research involving more than minimal risk, an explanation as to whether any compensation and an explanation as to whether any medical treatments are available if injury occurs, and if so, what they consist of, or where further information may be obtained.
7. An explanation of whom to contact for answers to pertinent questions about the research and research subjects' rights, and whom to contact in the event of a research-related injury to the subject.
8. A statement that participation is voluntary, that refusal to participate will involve no penalty or loss of benefits to which the subject is otherwise entitled, and that the subject may discontinue participation at any time without penalty or loss of benefits to which the subject is otherwise entitled.

Additional Elements of Informed Consent
1. A statement that the particular treatment or procedure may involve risks to the subject (or embryo or fetus, if the subject is or may become pregnant) which are currently unforeseeable.
2. Anticipated circumstances under which the subject's participation may be terminated by the investigator without regard to the subject's consent.
3. Any additional costs to the subject that may result from participation in the research.
4. The consequences of a subject's decision to withdraw from the research and procedures for orderly termination of participation by the subject.
5. A statement that significant new findings developed during the course of the research which may relate to the subject's willingness to continue participation will be provided to the subject.
6. The approximate number of subjects involved in the study.

Note. From 21 C.F.R. § 50.25 (2014). Retrieved from http://www.accessdata.fda.gov/scripts/cdrh/cfdocs/cfCFR/CFRSearch.cfm?CFRPart=50&showFR=1.

curriculum, revisions to the informed consent template, and a toolbox. The tool-box would be used by research staff, upon approval by the IRB, for studies that may be too complex to understand. Tools could include a one-page summary, schedule of events, contact information of a participant advocate, and a capacity evaluation tool (Palmer, 2013). In true circumstances where understanding is not possible, use of a legally authorized representative, a shortened version of the consent form, or other measures as indicated or stipulated by the IRB may be appropriate. In addition, federal regulations also require the IRB to have people review the study who have specific expertise related to identifiable vulnerable groups, such as pediatricians for studies involving children (21 C.F.R. § 56.107).

As patient advocates, nurses need to ensure that the consent process is truly voluntary and without coercion. Providing the required information alone is not enough. Ample time must be allowed for meaningful opportunities to engage in critical reflection concerning values and whether decision-making processes are enhanced or hindered by other factors. Bell and Ho (2011) discussed several social factors that can undermine the authenticity of the consent process. Some patients may not act voluntarily because of fear of consequences or the desire to please their family, friends, or physicians. Discussing decisions with others is not necessarily problematic; however, it is important to carefully assess patients' reasons for participating to ensure that they are acting according to their own values and preferences.

Placebos

When considering participation in a clinical trial, many patients fear receiving a placebo in place of active treatment. Placebos can be used in clinical trials, but only when there is no known recommended or standard treatment (van der Graaf & van Delden, 2009). According to Chambers (2011), for the state of equipoise to exist, participants should not be randomized to conditions when it is believed that better alternatives exist. Experimental treatments must be at least comparable to the standard of care as a precondition to offering participation in clinical trials. If an effective treatment exists, then the experimental treatment would be compared to the known or current standard. The beneficence principle of the Belmont Report dictates that there must always be an attempt to maximize possible benefits and minimize possible harms (National Commission for the Protection of Human Subjects of Biomedical and Behavioral Research, 1979). To offer a participant something below standard or to withhold known effective treatment would be unethical.

Confidentiality

Throughout the clinical trial process, a plethora of medical information is collected and submitted to the sponsor. In cancer research, specimens are frequently collected and analyzed for genetic information. This can be viewed as a risk to subjects for fear of possible discrimination in obtaining or maintaining employment or insurance coverage. Laws such as the Genetic Information Nondiscrimination Act and the Patient Protection and Affordable Care Act make it illegal for these data to be used to refuse employment (U.S. Equal Employment Opportunity Commission, 2008) or insurance (U.S. Department of Health and Human Services, 2010), but the possibility of disclosure may persuade a subject not to participate. The information that will be collected, used, and shared must be communicated with potential participants. As 21 C.F.R. § 56.111 states, adequate provisions to protect the privacy of the participants and to maintain the confidentiality of data must be in place. Under the HIPAA Privacy Rule (45 C.F.R. § 164.502), a covered entity may use or disclose de-identified health information for research purposes if the subject has given authorization (U.S. Department of Health and Human Services, 2013). When information is submitted, personal identifiers are removed or obliterated and usually only a study number and patient initials remain. The rule also requires that subjects be informed of uses and disclosures of their medical information for research purposes, as well as their rights to access their information. These rules help to ensure participants' privacy and the confidentiality of information. It is the responsibility of nurses and other healthcare personnel to respect these rules and inform participants of their rights and how their information is protected.

Implications Beyond the Research Subject

Ethics in research does not just apply to the individual research subject. The main purpose of research is to add to the general body of scientific knowledge, thereby improving health care for society (National Commission for the Protection of Human Subjects of Biomedical and Behavioral Research, 1979). This purpose cannot be fulfilled if the study has a poor research design or unreliable findings. The integrity of a study not only affects the individual participant but also can have far-reaching effects on the health care of others. Many of the decisions made during a study ultimately affect society as a whole. How data are collected, reported, and eventually published translates into how a given health problem will be addressed by clinicians in the future. New therapies may come to market that are ineffective or even unsafe when protocols are not adhered to, toxicity information is not collected or reported correctly, or results are published prematurely. This not only harms the trust that society has in the research community, but it also unnecessarily uses study subjects without adding any value to the improvement of health care.

Implications for Nursing Practice

Cancer is considered a serious health problem, with 1,658,210 new cases and 595,690 deaths estimated to occur in 2016 in the United States (Siegel, Miller,

& Jemal, 2016). With these statistics, it is not uncommon for oncology nurses to care for patients who are considering or participating in a clinical trial. Patient advocacy, documentation, and communication with the research team all contribute to the ethical conduct and safety of a clinical trial.

The significance of patient advocacy in research is critical to ensure adherence to all ethical principles in research and elements of the ethical codes (Hardicre, 2014; Sims, 2010). The third provision of the American Nurses Association's (2015) *Code of Ethics for Nurses* states, "The nurse promotes, advocates for, and protects the rights, health, and safety of the patient" (p. 9). This statement is fundamental to research and congruent with the ethical principles of the Belmont Report.

Acting as advocates, nurses listen to and support patients during their consideration of clinical trial participation. Several studies have demonstrated that many subjects, although they felt they were adequately informed, had unrealistic expectations of benefits and did not understand the nature and risk of participation (Beadle, Mengersen, Moynihan, & Yates, 2011; Behrendt, Gölz, Roesler, Bertz, & Wünsch, 2011; Joffe, Cook, Cleary, Clark, & Weeks, 2001; Meneguin & Ayres, 2014). It is not uncommon for patients with cancer to be motivated by the hope of physical benefit when faced with limited treatment options. Beliefs and attitudes are important influences on their decisions (Beadle et al., 2011). Nurses are key in assisting patients in setting realistic expectations and making the study details clear enough for them to make an autonomous decision on whether to participate.

Caring for patients in clinical trials requires comprehensive assessment, accurate documentation, and various reporting requirements. It is frequently the clinical trial nurses who communicate and coordinate protocol requirements. However, every healthcare team member is responsible for adhering to protocols and regulations in order to protect all study subjects. Frequently, patients may inform the nurse of certain side effects but fail to share these with the physician or the research team. Research protocols incorporate safety features to hold, reduce, or stop treatment if certain conditions occur. Early stopping rules may also be in place to terminate the entire study for certain conditions. Failure to report these in an expeditious fashion could have safety implications for all participants in the study. Therefore, it is important to document side effects accurately and discuss them with the study team (Sims, 2010).

Patients with cancer who are faced with limited options are at risk for exploitation (Beadle et al., 2011). Many factors can influence a clinician's judgment and challenge ethical conduct during a clinical trial. Some of these can include a conflict of interest, such as financial support or prestige within the scientific community. Nurses need to be watchful for and cognizant of the vulnerability of research subjects to protect them from harm and exploitation (Sims, 2010). It is important for nurses to know whom to contact to discuss possible concerns. The first place to start would be with the principal investigator of the study. If the concern remains unresolved, the IRB or the institution's human research protection officer can provide guidance.

Case Study

Jessica Thompson is a 63-year-old woman with stage I adenocarcinoma of the lung. She is married and has two adult children and a very supportive husband. Mrs. Thompson was diagnosed two months ago and has undergone a curative resection of the tumor. She presents to an oncologist, Dr. Raepy, as part of her multidisciplinary evaluation. Dr. Raepy is a prominent investigator at his institution, with many grants and sponsorships from pharmaceutical companies. He also has a keen interest in lung cancer and is part owner of a patent for an investigational device that can identify specific genetic mutations in cancer cells.

Mrs. Thompson expresses she is not sure why she needs to see an oncologist, as the surgeon informed her that he "got it all" and that she is cured. The oncologist explains that although there may not be any visible cancer, a cure cannot be guaranteed this early. He further explains that the current standard of care for stage I lung cancer after surgery is to watch and wait. However, there is a clinical trial that she could participate in to potentially decrease the chances of her cancer coming back.

The clinical trial consists of submission of tumor tissue to identify if there are specific molecular mutations that can be targeted by a new drug that is being evaluated. If Mrs. Thompson has the mutation and wishes to participate, she will be randomized to the investigational agent or a placebo for a period of one year. The study also requires continued medical visits, including blood draws, computed tomography scans, and physician visits. The oncologist explains this to Mrs. Thompson and adds that because the agent is an oral pill and targets the specific mutation on the tumor, it is generally better tolerated than chemotherapy.

Mrs. Thompson attended this appointment alone, as she did not feel that any treatment was going to be discussed. She requests that Dr. Raepy give her time to discuss this with her husband. The physician agrees but requests an answer within the week, as only so many openings are left in the study. He gives her the consent form and makes a follow-up appointment to sign the consent and submit her tissue.

At her next visit, Mrs. Thompson and her husband are met by the research nurse. The nurse asks Mrs. Thompson and her husband if they have any questions related to the study and what their thoughts are. Mrs. Thompson shares that she really does not want to participate in a clinical trial because she was told she was cured. In addition, her husband shares that Mrs. Thompson has had hearing loss related to Ménière disease, which also affects her balance at times. It is stated in the informed consent that the investigational agent can decrease hearing and may have other neurologic effects. The nurse explains that as long as Mrs. Thompson is able to conduct her activities of daily living, this would not exclude her from the study; however, aggravation of the Ménière disease is a potential risk. Mrs. Thompson states that she is willing to let them test her tissue to see if the mutation is present, but she really does not want to be in the study if she has to get the investigational agent. The research nurse explains that the results of the tumor testing would not be shared with her and that she cannot choose which treatment to get. Mrs. Thompson and her husband request to talk with Dr. Raepy.

Dr. Raepy discusses Mrs. Thompson's concerns and states that there is currently no evidence of Ménière disease being affected by this agent and that he has not found neurologic changes in other participants. He also informs her that if problems do occur, she is free to discontinue participation in the study. After much discussion, Mrs. Thompson agrees to participate in the study. Dr. Raepy then calls back the research nurse to obtain Mrs. Thompson's consent.

Discussion

Several ethical issues are present in this scenario. One needs to first question if a conflict of interest exists with this investigator and the trial. Conflicts of interest, if they exist, are to be disclosed and managed. If this is a federally funded study, any conflict of interest would need to be disclosed through the sponsoring agency and to the IRB of record. When a situation exists that can cloud the judgment of an investigator or other healthcare personnel, patients need to be informed. Another investigator without a conflict of interest should perhaps be responsible for obtaining the consent of participants. How this is handled would be explained within the local IRB's standard operating procedures.

The issue of the patient being told she is cured by the surgeon is not uncommon. Whether true or not, explaining this to the patient is not unethical. However, the statement that participation in a clinical trial can reduce the chances of the cancer returning is misleading. This is not clinical equipoise on the part of the doctor. Only half of the patients will receive the investigational drug. Even if it does decrease recurrence, the patient may not receive this agent. Moreover, the study is research; it is unknown if the treatment will truly work.

The discussion related to the toleration of the agent could also be misleading. Although many targeted agents may be tolerated differently than chemotherapy, side effects still can occur. When discussing side effects with patients, study personnel must not minimize the effects. These misleading statements undermine the ethical principles that surround informed consent. Without full and accurate information, a patient cannot make an autonomous decision.

In this case, the investigator may be coercing the subject into participation. Mrs. Thompson is given time to review the consent with her significant other; however, her concerns related to side effects are not well addressed. In research, there are many unknowns related to concurrent medical conditions. One cannot say with certainty that there will be no side effects, especially in this case when the agent is known to affect the nervous system. As stated in the Belmont Report, "To respect autonomy is to give weight to autonomous persons' considered opinions and choices while refraining from obstructing their actions unless they are clearly detrimental to others" (National Commission for the Protection of Human Subjects of Biomedical and Behavioral Research, 1979).

As a patient advocate, the research nurse needs to support the patient's decision and clarify her understanding of the risks and benefits of the study. The research nurse should not obtain the patient's consent without having further discussion with the investigator or IRB.

Conclusion

Many ethical principles guide researchers while conducting a study. These principles, founded within the Belmont Report and other documents, serve as a foundation for the conduct of ethical research. Federal regulations are based on these works and give a legal framework that honors these ethical principles. History has demonstrated that without these rules, the best interests of study subjects are often neglected. As advocates, nurses have a moral obligation to protect patients, lest past atrocities repeat. Nurses need to go beyond just following the rules and internalize the spirit of the regulations into their practice.

References

American Nurses Association. (2015). *Code of ethics for nurses with interpretive statements.* Retrieved from http://www.nursingworld.org/MainMenuCategories/EthicsStandards/CodeofEthicsforNurses/Code-of-Ethics-For-Nurses.html

Beadle, G., Mengersen, K., Moynihan, S., & Yates, P. (2011). Perceptions of the ethical conduct of cancer trials by oncology nurses. *European Journal of Cancer Care, 20,* 585–592. doi:10.1111/j.1365-2354.2011.01251.x

Beecher, H.K. (1966). Ethics and clinical research. *New England Journal of Medicine, 274,* 1354–1360. doi:10.1056/NEJM196606162742405

Behrendt, C., Gölz, T., Roesler, C., Bertz, H., & Wünsch, A. (2011). What do our patients understand about their trial participation? Assessing patients' understanding of their informed consent consultation about randomized clinical trials. *Journal of Medical Ethics, 37,* 74–80. doi:10.1136/jme.2010.035485

Bell, J., & Ho, A. (2011). Authenticity as a necessary condition for voluntary choice: A case study in cancer clinical trial participation. *American Journal of Bioethics, 11*(8), 33–35. doi:10.1080/15265 161.2011.583330

Cadeddu, M., Farrokhyar, F., Thoma, A., Haines, T., Garnett, A., & Goldsmith, C.H. (2008). Users' guide to the surgical literature: How to assess power and sample size. *Canadian Journal of Surgery, 51,* 476–482.

Chambers, D.W. (2011). Confusions in the equipoise concept and the alternative of fully informed overlapping rational decisions. *Medicine, Health Care and Philosophy, 14,* 133–142. doi:10.1007/s11019-010-9255-2

Cohen, J. (1988). *Statistical power analysis for the behavioral sciences* (2nd ed.). Hillsdale, NJ: Lawrence Erlbaum Associates.

Emanuel, E.J., Wendler, D., & Grady, C. (2000). What makes clinical research ethical? *JAMA, 283,* 2701–2711. doi:10.1001/jama.283.20.2701

Hardicre, J. (2014). An overview of research ethics and learning from the past. *British Journal of Nursing, 23,* 483–486. doi:10.12968/bjon.2014.23.9.483

Hornblum, A.M., Newman, J.L., & Dober, G.J. (2013). *Against their will: The secret history of medical experimentation on children in Cold War America.* New York, NY: Palgrave Macmillan.

Jansen, L. (2009). The ethics of altruism in clinical research. *Hastings Center Report, 39*(4), 26–36. doi:10.1353/hcr.0.0164

Joffe, S., Cook, E.F., Cleary, P.D., Clark, J.W., & Weeks, J.C. (2001). Quality of informed consent in cancer clinical trials: A cross-sectional survey. *Lancet, 358,* 1772–1777. doi:10.1016/S0140 -6736(01)06805-2

Liu, M.B., & Davis, K. (2010). *A clinical trials manual from the Duke Clinical Research Institute: Lessons from a horse named Jim* (2nd ed.). Hoboken, NJ: Wiley-Blackwell.

McNeilly, P.J. (2011, September). *The genesis of the human subjects' protections, regulations, and biomedical research in the 21st century.* CDER Small Business Assistance Training Clinical Trial Workshop. Retrieved from http://www.fda.gov/downloads/Drugs/NewsEvents/UCM275441.pdf

Meneguin, S., & Ayres, J.A. (2014). Perception of the informed consent form by participants in clinical trials. *Investigación y Educación en Enfermería, 32,* 97–102. doi:10.1590/S0120 -53072014000100011

National Cancer Institute. (2014, December). NCI's clinical trials programs and initiatives. Retrieved from http://www.cancer.gov/research/areas/clinical-trials

National Cancer Institute Cancer Therapy Evaluation Program. (2013, May 12). NCI informed consent template. Retrieved from http://ctep.cancer.gov/protocolDevelopment/informed_consent. htm

National Commission for the Protection of Human Subjects of Biomedical and Behavioral Research. (1979, April 18). *The Belmont Report: Ethical principles and guidelines for the protection of human subjects of research.* Retrieved from http://www.hhs.gov/ohrp/policy/belmont.html

Nuremberg Code. (1949). In *Trials of war criminals before the Nuremberg military tribunals under Control Council Law No. 10.* (Vol. 2, pp. 181–182). Retrieved from http://www.loc.gov/rr/frd/ Military_Law/pdf/NT_war-criminals_Vol-II.pdf

Oncology Nursing Society. (2010). *Oncology clinical trials nurse competencies.* Retrieved from https:// www.ons.org/sites/default/files/ctncompetencies.pdf

Palmer, D. (2013). An evaluation of participants' understanding of the informed consent process. *Monitor, 27*(5), 9–12.

Parascandola, M. (2000). The history of clinical research in the United States. *SoCRA Source, 26,* 31–44.

Parker, C. (2010). The moral primacy of the human being. *Journal of Medical Ethics, 36,* 563–566. doi:10.1136/jme.2010.037390

Sachs, B. (2009). Going from principles to rules in research ethics. *Bioethics, 25*(1), 9–20. doi:10.1111/ j.1467-8519.2009.01744.x

Sargent, D. (2014, May 5). *The role of statistics in cancer research* [Webinar]. Retrieved from https:// www.allianceforclinicaltrialsinoncology.org/main/cmsfile?cmsPath=/Public/Annual%20 Meeting/files/Role%20of%20Statistics%20in%20Cancer%20Research%20.pdf

Saunders, C. (1995). From involuntary subject to invited participant: The evolving consent process. *Research Nurse, 1*(6), 21–28.

Schlichting, D.E. (2010). Destabilizing the 'equipoise' framework in clinical trials: Prioritizing non-exploitation as an ethical framework in clinical research. *Nursing Philosophy, 11,* 271–279. doi:10.1111/j.1466-769X.2010.00455.x

Siegel, R.L., Miller, K.D., & Jemal, A. (2016). Cancer statistics, 2016. *CA: A Cancer Journal for Clinicians, 66,* 7–30. doi:10.3322/caac.21332

Sims, J.M. (2010). A brief review of the Belmont Report. *Dimensions of Critical Care Nursing, 29,* 173–174. doi:10.1097/DCC.0b013e3181de9ec5

21 C.F.R. pt. 50 (2014). Retrieved from http://www.accessdata.fda.gov/scripts/cdrh/cfdocs/cfCFR/ CFRSearch.cfm?CFRPart=50&showFR=1

21 C.F.R. pt. 56 (2014). Retrieved from http://www.accessdata.fda.gov/scripts/cdrh/cfdocs/cfCFR/ CFRSearch.cfm?CFRPart=56&showFR=1

Ubel, P.A., & Silbergleit, R. (2011). Behavioral equipoise: A way to resolve ethical stalemates in clinical research. *American Journal of Bioethics, 11*(2), 1–8. doi:10.1080/15265161.2010.540061

U.S. Department of Health and Human Services. (2010). The Affordable Care Act. Retrieved from http://www.hhs.gov/healthcare/rights/law/index.html

U.S. Department of Health and Human Services. (2013). Health information privacy. Retrieved from http://www.hhs.gov/ocr/privacy/hipaa/understanding/special/research

U.S. Equal Employment Opportunity Commission. (2008, May). The Genetic Information Nondiscrimination Act of 2008. Retrieved from http://eeoc.gov/laws/statutes/gina.cfm

van der Graaf, R., & van Delden, J. (2009). What is the best standard for the standard of care in clinical research? *American Journal of Bioethics, 9*(3), 35–43. doi:10.1080/15265160802654129

World Medical Association. (1996). Declaration of Helsinki. *BMJ, 313,* 1448–1449. doi:10.1136/bmj.313.7070.1448a

World Medical Association. (2013). Declaration of Helsinki. Retrieved from http://www.wma.net/en/30publications/10policies/b3/index.html

CHAPTER 3

Treatment Decision Making

Randy A. Jones, PhD, RN, FAAN, and Cathy Campbell, PhD, RN

Introduction

Each person with cancer and his or her caregivers will be cared for by oncology nurses who participate in the delivery of cancer therapy, educate patients and families, manage symptoms and side effects, and serve as patient advocates (McLennon, Uhrich, Lasiter, Chamness, & Helft, 2013). As members of interprofessional teams, nurses have complex and challenging roles (Bakker et al., 2013; Pavlish, Brown-Saltzman, Hersh, Shirk, & Nudelman, 2011; Ulrich et al., 2010). In these complex roles, nurses often face ethical issues in practice, especially in treatment decision making.

The majority of cancers develop in older adults, with 78% of cases being diagnosed in people aged 55 and older (American Cancer Society, 2015). The National Institute on Aging has reported a dramatic increase in average life expectancy, which may translate into more people being diagnosed with noncommunicable diseases such as diabetes, heart disease, and cancer (National Institute on Aging, 2011). As of January 1, 2014, an estimated 14.5 million cancer survivors were alive in the United States, and 72% of those survivors were 60 years of age or older (DeSantis et al., 2014). As people live longer and are more at risk of being diagnosed with multiple chronic and often life-threatening diseases, difficult issues frequently emerge related to decision making in cancer treatment.

Treatment decision making has become a focus of attention over the past four decades. Before the 1970s, treatment decisions were typically made by healthcare providers, excluding patients from being actively involved in informed and shared treatment decision making (Smith, Flamm, & Pentz, 2009). At this time, health care followed predominantly a paternalistic model in which healthcare providers made decisions for patients, often without involving them. This was because of healthcare providers' beliefs that patients could not understand the complexities of treatment decisions and that they would consider patients' best interests (Coulter, 2011). In this model, the control in the healthcare provider–patient relationship rested with the healthcare provider instead of the patient, and the patient played a more passive role. Multiple factors have contributed to a shift away from paternalistic decision making toward a model where decision making is a shared process between healthcare providers and patients.

In 2001, the Institute of Medicine report *Crossing the Quality Chasm* called for a redesign of health care, with attention focused on "patient-centered care" where healthcare decisions are guided by each patient's preferences, needs, and values. As medical science advanced, more treatment options became available as reasonable choices for various diseases. Society began to emphasize individual freedoms and rights, especially the rights of patients as consumers of health care. Patients began desiring more information from their healthcare providers so they could participate in and take responsibility for the decisions that were best for them, based on their personal values and preferences (Eldh, Ekman, & Ehnfors, 2006; Smith et al., 2009).

Dy and Purnell (2012) identified key concepts that must be present in the patient–provider encounter for quality, shared decision making to occur. Healthcare providers must be competent and trustworthy, and information about the disease and options must be current, accurate, and evidence based. Information must be effectively communicated between the patient and the healthcare team in a way that respects the cultural background, experience, and level of understanding of each unique patient and family. (See Chapter 6 for a full discussion about communication.) Relevant patient-centered concepts include the patient's capacity or competence to make decisions and/or the presence of a surrogate or healthcare proxy who is able to reliably and competently make decisions for the patient, based on the patient's preferences. In addition, the context of the scenario influences how involved patients want to be and should be when making a treatment decision. For example, in particularly urgent and critical situations, patients may follow physician recommendations rather than preferring to make these decisions for themselves.

In addition to respecting patients' right to choose their own health care, shared decision making in multiple healthcare settings has the potential to achieve other positive outcomes, including an increased use of beneficial interventions, reductions in the use of interventions not associated with clear benefits, and enhanced adherence to evidence-based recommendations for practice (Légaré et al., 2010). Despite these benefits, however, the shift to shared decision making has its own barriers from both the patient and healthcare provider viewpoints. Patient barriers to shared decision making include poor literacy, lack of assertiveness, and distress at the time of illness, which can prevent patients from being fully informed and able to participate in a comprehensive discussion of treatment options. Healthcare providers also find barriers to shared decision making with patients. In a systematic review of evidence, Gravel, Légaré, and Graham (2006) found that the most cited barrier to shared decision making by healthcare providers is time constraint. Studies have found that healthcare providers want patients to participate in their care, but patients need time to absorb the impact of diagnosis before making treatment decisions. Healthcare providers feel they have an insufficient amount of time to spend with patients, especially when discussing difficult treatment decisions. They may face additional barriers related to patients' competency and cultural characteristics.

While physicians and other primary care providers lead most discussions with patients about decisions related to cancer treatment, oncology nurses are often in positions to provide support and clarification to patients about treatment information, to advocate for patients' rights and values, and to intervene when they identify limitations in the shared decision-making process. Because ethical issues in treatment decision making are vast and complicated, a consideration of ethical principles may help nurses and other healthcare professionals through these difficult situations. This chapter will address selected topics related to shared decision making that raise ethical issues, discuss implications for nursing practice, and provide an illustration of shared decision making using a case study.

Ethical Principles Related to Decision Making

Four ethical principles that relate specifically to nursing practice and decision making are respect for autonomy, veracity, justice (distributive), and beneficence. Respect for autonomy is central when nurses and other healthcare professionals think about decision making. The main consideration under this principle is respecting and protecting patient and family rights, values, and preferences during the decision-making process (Beauchamp & Childress, 2012; Ulrich et al., 2010). Also important is encouraging and advocating for patients to have and use the necessary resources to make free and informed decisions based on their abilities, culture, and values. Closely related to autonomy in this context is the principle of veracity. Beauchamp and Childress (2012) referred to veracity as the comprehensive and accurate delivery of health information. Healthcare providers need the clinical expertise, knowledge, and skills to be able to communicate relevant and up-to-date information about the disease and treatment options to each patient and family. The effective delivery of health information is influenced by patients' health literacy level and ability to communicate through speaking, listening, reading, and writing. Next, distributive justice is an important ethical principle to ensure that every person has equal access to shared decision making about their treatment, especially as the world begins to see how the Patient Protection and Affordable Care Act will transform access to care as well as treatment decisions in the United States. Significant racial, ethnic, and geographic health disparities in the availability of health care have been well documented (McWilliams, 2009; McWilliams, Meara, Zaslavsky, & Ayanian, 2007). Despite the many advances that have been made in cancer treatment, patients who are members of certain racial and ethnic groups and those living in rural communities may not have adequate access to cancer care or to the full range of treatment options. Finally, beneficence is one of the principles salient to any discussion of decision making. Healthcare providers aim to provide information and involve patients in decision making in helpful and supportive ways. They aim to offer treatment options that will optimize patient outcomes in terms of quality and quantity of life and minimize harm and cost. However, these positive outcomes and the cost-benefit ratio are not always easily determined by healthcare providers nor understood by patients and families.

Ethical Issues Related to Shared Decision Making

Making decisions about life-saving or life-altering cancer therapy is complex, and patients can feel overwhelmed when asked to participate in choosing a therapeutic treatment option. Within treatment decision making, challenging areas that often raise ethical issues include (a) patient characteristics that compromise autonomy and participation in decision making, and (b) providing accurate and honest information to guide decisions to change or stop treatment. Oncology nurses may commonly experience these situations in clinical practice and witness how the principles of autonomy, veracity, justice, fidelity, and beneficence, among others, are compromised, causing distress for patients, their families, and the healthcare team. The following discussion will provide some context for these issues and highlight their importance.

Patient Characteristics That Compromise Autonomy

The American Nurses Association's (2015) *Code of Ethics for Nurses* emphasizes respect for the individual and primacy of the nurse–patient relationship, understanding that the patient may be an individual, family, or community. Regardless of clinical specialty area or healthcare setting, at the source of the most ethical challenges or dilemmas in clinical practice are conflicts over respect for the individual, such as protecting the patient's rights and informed consent for treatments and procedures (Cohen & Erickson, 2006; McLennon et al., 2013; Ulrich et al., 2010).

When deciding to start cancer treatment, information provided to a patient or surrogate during the informed consent process prior to any procedure or medical treatment includes basic information about the cancer and condition, purpose of the treatment, alternative options, and expected side effects and risks (Berg, Appelbaum, Lidz, & Parker, 2001; Workman, 2013). Physicians (and advanced practice nurses, in some settings) prescribe cancer therapy and obtain the informed consent from patients, their surrogates, or other legally authorized representatives. Increasingly, surrogates may be long-distance caregivers (Gouin, Glaser, Malarkey, Beversdorf, & Kiecolt-Glaser, 2012) who are providing consent to authorize treatments via the phone, fax, or Internet. The healthcare provider who meets with the patient, surrogate, and other caregivers must evaluate the patient's competence, freedom from coercion, and understanding of the risks, benefits, and options of the potential treatment or procedure.

Patients receiving cancer treatments may not always have a full understanding of the treatment planned and the expected side effects because of factors such as treatment-related anxiety, a decline in physical and cognitive status related to medications and other treatments, and the physiologic impact of the cancer (Beauchamp & Childress, 2012; Bender, Ergÿn, Rosenzweig, Cohen, & Sereika, 2005), such as brain metastasis or hypercalcemia (Seccareccia, 2010). Other barriers to the informed consent process include the lack of general and health-specific literacy for patients who do and do not speak, read, or understand English (Friedman, Corwin, Dominick, & Rose, 2009; Kilbridge et al., 2009; Scheier, 2009; Thomas & Collier, 2009).

According to the National Assessment of Adult Literacy (NAAL) (Kutner, Greenberg, Jin, & Paulsen, 2006), approximately 36% of adults in the United States have limited health literacy, 22% have basic health literacy, and 14% have below basic health literacy. When race is considered, NAAL found that Caucasians score better on health literacy when compared to other ethnic or racial groups (i.e., African Americans, Hispanics, Asians, and Native Americans). Studies have associated low literacy skills with poor health outcomes (Berkman et al., 2011; Kutner et al., 2006). Berkman et al. (2011) found that individuals with lower health literacy had an increase in hospitalizations, greater emergency care use, and lower use of mammography, along with a higher risk of mortality for older adults. Several studies have shown that minority patients may be less responsive and less participatory than Caucasian patients when interacting with Caucasian healthcare providers (Johnson, Roter, Powe, & Cooper, 2004; Peek et al., 2010). In the study by Peek and colleagues (2010), African American patients with diabetes reported several race-related issues that affected decision-making behaviors, such as a power imbalance, negative attitudes toward Caucasian physicians, and a likelihood to defer to the physician.

Patients with low levels of health literacy encounter challenges in the satisfactory access and utilization of health care as well as provider–patient interactions, including decision making (Friedman et al., 2009; Kilbridge et al., 2009). Kilbridge and colleagues (2009), for example, found that in a sample of primarily low-income, rural-dwelling African American men, even the patients who had received treatment for prostate cancer did not recognize important anatomic structures or terms related to possible side effects of prostate cancer treatment, such as erection, impotence, and incontinence. Surprisingly, 95% of the total sample did not recognize the word *incontinence*. An understanding of erection, impotence, and incontinence would be needed to fully understand the benefits, risks, and side effects of prostate cancer–related treatments, such as prostatectomy, radiation therapy, and antiandrogen therapy (Kilbridge et al., 2009; Liebertz & Fox, 2006).

By its very nature, the process of medical decision making is emotionally laden and at times can be filled with uncertainty for patients and their caregivers. The intensity of decision-making context is exacerbated by premorbid psychological distress, such as depression and anxiety, emotional distress as a side effect of cancer-related treatment, and the expression of grief for actual or potential losses (Gil, Costa, Hilker, & Benito, 2012; Thekkumpurath, Venkateswaran, Kumar, Newsham, & Bennett, 2009).

Teunissen, de Graeff, Voest, and de Haes (2007) found that 29% of the participants in their study of hospitalized patients had anxiety and depression as comorbid conditions. Anxiety and depression can negatively affect key components in the decision-making process, including expressing personal values, interpreting risk estimates, problem solving, and considering possibilities beyond current circumstances such as intense symptom distress (i.e., pain or fatigue) (Power, Swartzman, & Robinson, 2011).

Once cancer treatment is initiated, treatment-related side effects may include cognitive and physical fatigue, emotional lability, and neurocognitive dysfunction (Liebertz & Fox, 2006). These side effects may interfere with or change the patient's ability to participate in making decisions. Depending on the urgency of the situation, decision making can be delayed or timed to coincide with periods of low symptom burden or to avoid periods of symptom exacerbation.

Finally, patients experience emotional distress related to the impact of the cancer diagnosis or reaction to any event along the trajectory (Power et al., 2011), including grief for actual or potential losses. Although grief and depression have different etiologies, some of the physical and behavioral indicators that influence decision making overlap, such as slower cognitive processing, sleep pattern disturbances, and difficulties with problem solving.

Providing Accurate and Honest Information to Guide Decision Making

The decision to change lines of therapy when the cancer is no longer responsive to the initial line of treatment can bring forth ethical issues. The importance of having adequate information and time to make an informed decision about a change in cancer treatment is imperative. Some patients with cancer may feel pressured by healthcare providers to have a particular treatment (Hall, Boyd, Lippert, & Theodorescu, 2003) or feel rushed to move to a second, third, or consequential cancer treatment (Ramfelt & Lützén, 2005). Gurmankin, Baron, Hershey, and Ubel (2002) found that healthcare providers may influence patients' treatment decisions to a degree that patients go against their own treatment preferences. Patients' treatment preferences may be different from their healthcare providers' recommendations. Patients may have prioritized other issues in their lives in addition to health improvement, such as working at a job or caring for family members, which healthcare providers may not necessarily think about because they have different beliefs about the course of the disease and treatment (Keirns & Goold, 2009). As patients may move to other lines of cancer treatment, it is important for healthcare providers to inform patients about the consequences of their choices and come to a treatment plan that is consistent with the patients' goals.

Patients and family members may feel that they want to maintain hope throughout treatment and that they must move forward with treatment if the initial treatment fails. One study showed that healthcare providers often overestimate prognosis by at least 30% (Glare et al., 2003), which can give patients a potentially false outlook on their treatment and health. There is a pressure of maintaining hope in the treatment that is felt by patients and their healthcare providers (Little & Sayers, 2004), which may make patients feel that they have little control in the decision-making process and must continue with the course trajectory.

Stopping cure-focused treatment is another critical decision in a declining disease trajectory. Not only is this decision a major turning point for patients and families (Campbell, Williams, & Orr, 2010), but it is also a source of ethical conflict for members of the interprofessional team, especially when the physical decline is accompanied by cognitive changes that may affect decision making (Cohen & Erickson, 2006; McLennon et al., 2013). Patients frequently receive cancer-related treatment very late in the disease course. Temel and colleagues (2010) found in a sample of patients with metastatic non-small cell lung cancer that 21% of patients received chemotherapy within 14 days of death and 36% received chemotherapy within 30 days of death. Nurses shared clinical narratives about giving chemotherapy to patients who are within hours to days of death (McLennon et al., 2013). Nurses are faced with multiple ethical dilemmas that may stem from institutional culture, family beliefs and wishes, and healthcare laws, as well as others. Decision making is quite complex, and those institutional, family, and societal norms may be perceived as barriers that can cause ethical tension for nurses.

Consistent with clinical narratives about administering chemotherapy to people with a life expectancy measured in days to weeks, hospice referrals are often delayed until the last weeks of life. Studies have shown that 30%–36% of people admitted to hospice die in seven days or less (Campbell, Baernholdt, Yan, Hinton, & Lewis, 2012; National Hospice and Palliative Care Organization [NHPCO], 2015), and the median length of stay in hospice programs in the United States is 17 days (NHPCO, 2015).

These conversations about changing the course of cancer treatment or stopping cancer-directed treatment are usually difficult and emotional situations for healthcare providers. Many physicians and nurses lack the communication skills and confidence for conveying difficult news to patients and families. These conversations, therefore, are often held too late in the course of illness or happen in such a way that adds to the patient's and family's emotional distress (Thorne,

Bultz, & Baile, 2005). Jangland, Gunningberg, and Carlsson (2009) reported that patients were dissatisfied and more anxious during treatment when they received inadequate information.

The cost of treatment not only can affect patients' financial situations but also takes a toll on their emotions, their time, and the lives of family members, friends, and coworkers. Out-of-pocket expenses play a major factor in how patients decide on their treatment, especially those of lower socioeconomic status. Langa et al. (2004) noted that individuals with low income may spend about 27% of their annual income on cancer treatment. The increasing financial strain on patients with cancer may create obstacles in receiving adequate health care in a timely manner, which becomes an ethical issue of fairness and justice, as defined by Beauchamp and Childress (2012). Those who are uninsured are more likely to be between the ages of 19 and 34 years, be Black or Hispanic, and work less than full time (DeNavas-Walt, Proctor, Smith, & U.S. Census Bureau, 2012). Because of the high cost of cancer care, many people may delay or forgo screening or treatment, resulting in uninsured individuals being more likely to be diagnosed with chronic disease and later-stage disease, less likely to survive the diagnosis, and more likely to have poorer health outcomes (McWilliams, 2009; McWilliams et al., 2007). Even when offered certain treatments, patients may forgo or delay that treatment to decrease cost (Kim, 2007). The exorbitant healthcare costs that patients experience at this vulnerable time increase their chances of debt and bankruptcy (Himmelstein, Warren, Thorne, & Woolhandler, 2005).

Healthcare providers may feel torn about whether to offer a treatment to a patient because of cost. Several studies have found that many healthcare providers are uncomfortable discussing cost with patients (Hardee, Platt, & Kasper, 2005; Schrag & Hanger, 2007). Neumann and colleagues (2010) found that 56% of oncologists agreed that cost influences what they recommend for cancer treatment to their patients. Healthcare providers believe cost is an important topic to discuss with patients, and patients do want to discuss cost with their healthcare providers; however, patients prefer that healthcare providers initiate the conversation (Alexander, Casalino, & Meltzer, 2003; Alexander, Casalino, Tseng, McFadden, & Meltzer, 2004). Barriers that impede open discussion of cost vary from both the patient and healthcare provider viewpoints (Meropol et al., 2009). Among healthcare providers, the most common barriers were insufficient time to discuss cost and not having a good solution to offer the patient. Patients may feel uncomfortable discussing cost with their healthcare providers and feel like they do not have enough time within the clinical setting. Patients may also believe that healthcare providers do not have a solution to their financial problems and are unsure what the impact of such discussion would have on their quality of care (Alexander et al., 2004).

Finally, shared decision making relies on healthcare providers conferring honest and accurate information about treatment options to patients and their families to match best practice recommendations with patient preferences and values. It is not uncommon, however, for situations to arise in the clinical setting where there is a lack of treatment options, a lack of evidence about the effectiveness of options, or true uncertainty about the course of disease (Braddock, 2013). Healthcare providers may feel conflicted about whether to acknowledge such uncertainty or lack of evidence for fear it may increase a patient's anxiety and distress and decrease trust and confidence in the provider–patient relationship.

Implications for Nursing Practice

As members of the interprofessional team, nurses play an important role in the shared decision-making process. In many settings, nurses are the healthcare providers most likely to have extended contact with patients and their family members. Prior to the start of treatment, the nurse can evaluate a patient's understanding of his or her cancer, the rationale for the planned treatment, and the short- and long-term side effects (Beauchamp & Childress, 2012). Although patients' understanding about their treatment is primary, attention should also be placed on patients who may have a surrogate. Surrogates need to understand the cancer treatment regimen, potential side effects, and other aspects of the patient's treatment for which they have given consent. Testing and feedback interventions are recommended that ask patients and their surrogates to repeat back in their own words what they understand about the planned treatment to ensure their understanding (Schenker, Fernandez, Sudore, & Schillinger, 2011).

Nurses are often responsible for carrying out the plan of care, including the administration of chemotherapy, other infusions, and medications and managing symptoms when interacting with patients across healthcare settings, ranging from inpatient acute care to ambulatory care and home care (Workman, 2013). As treatments continue, nurses protect patients' rights by ensuring that patients and surrogates remain informed throughout treatment. Informed consent is a process. Given that many cancer treatments produce side effects with long-term sequelae, such as the possibility of secondary cancers, infertility (Workman, 2013), cognitive changes (Bender et al., 2006; Workman, 2013), and permanent damage to major organs (Viale & Yamamoto, 2008), the need for ongoing discussion, supplemented with written materials and Internet-based resources, about treatment plans takes on greater significance (Schenker et al., 2011).

Nurses respect patient autonomy by being patient advocates, by understanding the values that underlie decision making, and by ensuring that organizations have structures in place to protect patient rights. Nurses can guide or support decision making more effectively by ensuring that patient education materials, consent forms, and decision aids address the needs of culturally diverse patients. Strategies should be put into place to ensure that all patients have the resources they need to participate in decisions about their own care (Schenker et al., 2011).

It is important for nurses and other healthcare providers to have an understanding of the complexity of the treatment decision-making process not only from the healthcare provider side, but also from the side of the patient and his or her support person. Patients are faced with a number of considerations including treatment costs, role changes in the family dynamics, the desires of family members, stigma of disease progression and treatment side effects, and other factors that affect how they make treatment decisions. Nurses can help sustain and improve the delivery of adequate treatment information to help patients feel satisfied with their treatment decisions by including support persons such as family and friends, who may play an important role in the decision-making process, particularly within African American families, who are more likely to engage in seeking informal advice to make decisions (Jones et al., 2010, 2011).

Cancer-related medical decision making can be negatively affected by a diagnosis of anxiety or depression antecedent to the cancer diagnosis, the emotional impact of cancer-related treatment as a side effect, or the reaction to the cancer diagnosis itself. Increasingly, cognitive behavioral interventions (CBIs) are being added to the plan of care to decrease emotional and psychological symptoms, to help with coping, and ultimately to support decision making during cancer treatment and along the survivorship journey. Advanced practice nurses, clinical psychologists, psychiatrists, and other licensed mental health counselors can provide CBIs (Breitbart et al., 2010; Campbell et al., 2012; Chambers, Pinnock, Lepore, Hughes, & O'Connell, 2011).

Community health workers and patient navigators are helpful team members to assist patients in understanding cancer treatment costs and seeking financial assistance for their treatment when necessary. They can help bridge the gap between the patient and healthcare provider/healthcare system to improve healthcare access. Because of many patients being uninsured and a belief that health insurance is an important part of receiving adequate health care, particularly among minorities such as African Americans (Jones et al., 2011), community health workers and patient navigators may be even more important. They could be particularly effective working with patients from minority populations who are diagnosed with cancer or undergoing cancer treatment (Wenzel, Jones, Klimmek, Szanton, & Krumm, 2012). Additionally, they can assist patient surrogates in finding more information about treatments and finding outside resources that may be available. This may help in allowing patients, particularly those who are minorities or with low socioeconomic status, to obtain fair and additional access to resources that may not be apparent. Other strategies to address the financial burden on patients and caregivers include educating and supporting healthcare providers about how to engage patients in discussions about treatment cost (Meropol et al., 2009).

Treatment decision making involves complex issues such as treatment side effects, previous healthcare experiences, and other considerations. As the number of cancer treatments steadily grows, an increased number of treatment options may be available for each patient, making the decision-making process more complex. Decision aids can be used to assist patients in applying certain health information and becoming active in the decision-making process (Stacey et al., 2014). Decision aids offer health information about various treatment options as well as strategies to help patients recognize the values they might place on various options and guidance about the steps in decision making. Decision aids are seen to be more effective when they are used in a shared decision-making process and in addition to counseling by healthcare providers (Skinner et al., 2004; Stacey et al., 2014). Studies have noted that the use of a decision aid that promotes a shared decision-making process between the healthcare provider, the patient, and the support person in the clinical setting seems to be appealing to patients and feasible in practice (Hajizadeh et al., 2013; Jones, Steeves, Ropka, & Hollen, 2013).

Allowing patients time to consider the options available with the appropriate information helps them to participate in treatment decision making (Ramfelt & Lützén, 2005). When clinical environments are rushed and time becomes a barrier that prevents the frequent and necessary conversations about treatment decisions, nurses and navigators can initiate discussions about shared decision making in the absence of the physician, who is usually the primary care provider. Thus, it is important to create a team culture with interprofessional practice values where all team members are working toward the same patient goals and outcomes.

Physicians, nurses, and other healthcare providers can improve their communication skills with continuing education and practice, especially to approach difficult conversations related to breaking bad news about a new cancer diagnosis, disease progression or recurrence, and the need to discontinue cancer treatments (Back et al., 2009). Continuing education programs that build communication skills are essential to improve the patient–healthcare provider relationship. Communication education programs and techniques (Back et al., 2009; Baile et al., 2000; Schapira, 2008) have been developed to improve healthcare providers' communication skills to increase patient satisfaction.

Even in situations where there is a lack of evidence or uncertainty about how to proceed, Braddock (2013) suggested that openly and honestly sharing information and decision making in this context can build trust and transparency between patients and the healthcare team. Open dialogues with opportunities for patients to learn what is and what is not known can be empowering and still contribute to their overall satisfaction.

Case Study

James Abrams is a retired 68-year-old African American man with recurrent prostate cancer after a prostatectomy two years ago. He had no high-risk features or cancer in his lymph nodes following surgery, so he has been followed by his oncology nurse practitioner (ONP) with regular monitoring of prostate-specific antigen (PSA) levels every six months. He has no family history of prostate cancer. His past medical history consists of diabetes mellitus, hypertension, and hypercholesterolemia, and his daily medications include lisinopril, atorvastatin calcium, and metformin. During this time off therapy, Mr. Abrams' PSA levels have been stable (0.8–1.1 ng/ml), and his only troubling symptom is erectile dysfunction. He is independent and leads an active lifestyle, attending weekly Bible study and church services and refurbishing his '68 Chevrolet. He is married and has two adult children and three grandchildren who live nearby.

Mr. Abrams returns to the clinic for a follow-up appointment with his soon-to-be retired wife and his daughter, who both accompany him to each clinic visit. During his appointment with the ONP, Mr. Abrams admits that he has been feeling more tired and has been less active than three months ago. He believes that the onset of his fatigue was associated with an upper respiratory infection several weeks earlier, but the fatigue has not fully resolved. The ONP notes that his blood counts and chemistry panels are normal but his PSA level has increased by 4.9 ng/ml. A computed tomography scan of his abdomen subsequently reveals two enlarged lymph nodes in the retroperitoneum that prove to be metastatic disease.

The ONP discusses the treatment options for recurrent cancer after prostatectomy with Mr. Abrams and his family. To help him make an informed decision about treatment, the ONP recommends use of a decision aid that includes written information as well as an interactive Internet program with videos and questionnaires. The decision aid outlines the benefits and side effects of the treatment options available to Mr. Abrams: (a) continue active surveillance with monitoring of PSA levels every three to six months; (b) begin androgen deprivation therapy with a luteinizing hormone-releasing hormone such as leuprolide; or (c) begin androgen deprivation therapy with a type of external beam radiation therapy. The ONP provides the written materials and demonstrates use of the website, which includes text and videos that describe each treatment option in detail, including how treatments are administered, side effects, the likelihood of cancer response, and estimated cost. The website also includes questions to help Mr. Abrams think about how he wants to be involved in making treatment decisions, how he wants to include his spouse, family, and friends in the decision, and what outcomes are most important to him, including survival outcomes, quality of life, and disease- or treatment-related symptoms. Mr. Abrams agrees to use the decision aid over the next two weeks and return for an appointment with the oncologist and ONP to determine the optimal treatment plan.

When Mr. Abrams returns to the clinic for his follow-up appointment with his wife and daughter, he states that he is feeling well and has spent quite a bit of time using the decision aid together with his wife on his home computer. In discussion with the oncologist and ONP, Mr. Abrams demonstrates a good understanding of the available treatment options as well as their benefits and risks. He states that he prefers and feels comfortable being an active participant in making a treatment decision. He has discussed his preferences with his wife and two other friends who have also been treated for prostate cancer. Mr. Abrams ultimately decides not to begin any treatment at the present time because he is feeling well and has a strong preference not to experience the side effects related to hormone therapy or radiation therapy, such as fatigue, hot flashes, and weight gain. In the next few months, he has plans to travel with his wife to celebrate her retirement and their anniversary. He states that he is comfortable with not initiating treatment for his cancer at this time, although he acknowledges that Mrs. Abrams worries about not starting treatment soon.

The oncologist and ONP support Mr. Abrams' decision not to begin any therapy at this time. Together they agree to continue to monitor his PSA levels every three months and consider revisiting this decision at each appointment based on his clinical condition and preferences. Mr. Abrams, his wife, and his daughter are satisfied with this decision.

Discussion

During times of difficult treatment decisions, healthcare providers must be able to recognize patients' and family members' priorities and information needs and allow them time to make those difficult decisions (Fowler, Levin, & Sepucha, 2011). A patient may be asking himself several questions, such as, "Should I start a treatment?" "Which treatment is best for me? I feel fine right now; should I wait a little longer?" "Will I disappoint my wife and daughter if I choose not to start treatment?" and "Will I be able to afford treatment if I decide to start it?" These questions and more may enter a patient's mind when faced with such complex and difficult healthcare decisions.

Family involvement plays a major role in how patients make decisions about their treatment. This is particularly common in the African American community, where patients are more likely to seek health advice from informal sources (Hamilton & Sandelowski, 2004; Jones, Steeves, & Williams, 2009). Prostate cancer is a disease that comes with physical and emotional effects. Because of the stigma that men with prostate cancer may face (e.g., issues related to incontinence and impotence), potential role changes in the family dynamics as a result of the man's diagnosis, and embarrassment, informal support systems may play a more critical part in the decision-making process, particularly among African Americans (Jones et al., 2010). Musa, Schulz, Harris, Silverman, and Thomas (2009) noted that African Americans are more likely to seek informal advice from family members, friends, and community members when compared to their Caucasian counterparts.

In the case study, the healthcare providers invited Mr. Abrams to actively participate in choosing the best treatment option for him based on evidence-based recommendations as well as his preferences and values. The use of the decision aid facilitated Mr. Abrams in understanding his treatment options, thinking about his preferred role in decision making, and recognizing what was most important for him and his family in order to make an informed and satisfying decision (Jones et al., 2013). Decision aids help patients and healthcare providers develop personalized decisions by focusing on options and outcomes related to the individual's healthcare situation (O'Connor et al., 2007; Stacey et al., 2011). They can be used to help patients apply specific health information while actively participating in health-related decision making and are most effective when tailored to individual patients and family members (Jones et al., 2013; Stacey et al., 2014).

Conclusion

The ethical concerns related to treatment decision making for cancer care are complicated, and patients and their families deserve time to understand the treatment options and make the best decision for their treatment. The ethical concerns related to shared decision making, especially when changing or stopping treatment, discussing cost, considering culture, and addressing uncertainty, are just a few of the dilemmas that may surface during the time of treatment decision-making. Patients have a number of treatment options for cancer that present different risks and benefits. Healthcare providers should be more aware that each patient has unique health beliefs that affect the ultimate decisions that are made. Decision aids and resources are available to help patients make well-informed, shared decisions about their treatment.

References

Alexander, G.C., Casalino, L.P., & Meltzer, D.O. (2003). Patient-physician communication about out-of-pocket costs. *JAMA, 290*, 953–958. doi:10.1001/jama.290.7.953

Alexander, G.C., Casalino, L.P., Tseng, C.W., McFadden, D., & Meltzer, D.O. (2004). Barriers to patient-physician communication about out-of-pocket costs. *Journal of General Internal Medicine, 19*, 856–860. doi:10.1111/j.1525-1497.2004.30249.x

American Cancer Society. (2015). *Cancer facts and figures 2015.* Retrieved from http://www.cancer.org/acs/groups/content/@editorial/documents/document/acspc-044552.pdf

American Nurses Association. (2015). *Code of ethics for nurses with interpretive statements.* Retrieved from http://www.nursingworld.org/MainMenuCategories/EthicsStandards/CodeofEthicsfor Nurses

Back, A.L., Arnold, R.M., Baile, W.F., Tulsky, J.A., Barley, G.E., Pea, R.D., & Fryer-Edwards, K.A. (2009). Faculty development to change the paradigm of communication skills teaching in oncology. *Journal of Clinical Oncology, 27*, 1137–1141. doi:10.1200/JCO.2008.20.2408

Baile, W.F., Buckman, R., Lenzi, R., Glober, G., Beale, E.A., & Kudelka, A.P. (2000). SPIKES—A six-step protocol for delivering bad news: Application to the patient with cancer. *Oncologist, 5*, 302–311. doi:10.1634/theoncologist.5-4-302

Bakker, D., Strickland, J., MacDonald, C., Butler, L., Fitch, M., Olson, K., & Cummings, G. (2013). The context of oncology nursing practice: An integrative review. *Cancer Nursing, 36*, 72–88. doi:10.1097/NCC.0b013e31824afadf

Beauchamp, T.L., & Childress, J.F. (2012). *Principles of biomedical ethics* (7th ed.). New York, NY: Oxford University Press.

Bender, C.M., Ergÿn, F.S., Rosenzweig, M.Q., Cohen, S.M., & Sereika, S.M. (2005). Symptom clusters in breast cancer across 3 phases of the disease. *Cancer Nursing, 28*, 219–225. doi:10.1097/00002820-200505000-00011

Bender, C.M., Sereika, S.M., Berga, S.L., Vogel, V.G., Brufsky, A.M., Paraska, K.K., & Ryan, C.M. (2006). Cognitive impairment associated with adjuvant therapy in breast cancer. *Psycho-Oncology, 15,* 422–430. doi:10.1002/pon.964

Berg, J.W., Appelbaum, P.S., Lidz, C.W., & Parker, L.S. (2001). *Informed consent: Legal theory and clinical practice* (2nd ed.). New York, NY: Oxford University Press.

Berkman, N., Sheridan, S., Donahue, K., Halpern, D., Viera, A., Crotty, K., … Viswanathan, M. (2011). *Health literacy interventions and outcomes: An updated systematic review* (Evidence Report/Technology Assessment No. 199). Rockville, MD: Agency for Healthcare Research and Quality.

Braddock, C.H., III. (2013). Supporting shared decision making when clinical evidence is low. *Medical Care Research and Review, 70*(Suppl. 1), 129S–140S. doi:10.1177/1077558712460280

Breitbart, W., Rosenfeld, B., Gibson, C., Pessin, H., Poppito, S., Nelson, C., … Olden, M. (2010). Meaning-centered group psychotherapy for patients with advanced cancer: A pilot randomized controlled trial. *Psycho-Oncology, 19,* 21–28. doi:10.1002/pon.1556

Campbell, C.L., Baernholdt, M., Yan, G., Hinton, I.D., & Lewis, E. (2012). Racial/ethnic perspectives on the quality of hospice care. *American Journal of Hospice and Palliative Medicine, 30,* 347–353. doi:10.1177/1049909112457455

Campbell, C.L., Williams, I.C., & Orr, T. (2010). Factors that impact end-of-life decision making in African Americans with advanced cancer. *Journal of Hospice and Palliative Nursing, 12,* 214–222. doi:10.1097/NJH.0b013e3181de1174

Chambers, S.K., Pinnock, C., Lepore, S.J., Hughes, S., & O'Connell, D.L. (2011). A systematic review of psychosocial interventions for men with prostate cancer and their partners. *Patient Education and Counseling, 85,* e75–e88. doi:10.1016/j.pec.2011.01.027

Cohen, J.S., & Erickson, J.M. (2006). Ethical dilemmas and moral distress in oncology nursing practice. *Clinical Journal of Oncology Nursing, 10,* 775–780. doi:10.1188/06.CJON.775-780

Coulter, A. (2011). *Engaging patients in healthcare.* New York, NY: Open University Press.

DeNavas-Walt, C., Proctor, B.D., Smith, J.C., & U.S. Census Bureau. (2012). *Income, poverty, and health insurance coverage in the United States: 2011* (No. P60-243). Washington, DC: U.S. Government Printing Office.

DeSantis, C.E., Lin, C.C., Mariotto, A.B., Siegel, R.L., Stein, K.D., Kramer, J.L., … Jemal, A. (2014). Cancer treatment and survivorship statistics, 2014. *CA: A Cancer Journal for Clinicians, 64,* 252–271. doi:10.3322/caac.21235

Dy, S.M., & Purnell, T.S. (2012). Key concepts relevant to quality of complex and shared decision-making in health care: A literature review. *Social Science and Medicine, 74,* 582–587. doi:10.1016/j.socscimed.2011.11.015

Eldh, A.C., Ekman, I., & Ehnfors, M. (2006). Conditions for patient participation and non-participation in health care. *Nursing Ethics, 13,* 503–514. doi:10.1191/0969733006nej898oa

Fowler, F.J., Jr., Levin, C.A., & Sepucha, K.R. (2011). Informing and involving patients to improve the quality of medical decisions. *Health Affairs, 30,* 699–706. doi:10.1377/hlthaff.2011.0003

Friedman, D.B., Corwin, S.J., Dominick, G.M., & Rose, I.D. (2009). African American men's understanding and perceptions about prostate cancer: Why multiple dimensions of health literacy are important in cancer communication. *Journal of Community Health, 34,* 449–460. doi:10.1007/s10900-009-9167-3

Gil, F., Costa, G., Hilker, I., & Benito, L. (2012). First anxiety, afterwards depression: Psychological distress in cancer patients at diagnosis and after medical treatment. *Stress and Health, 28,* 362–367. doi:10.1002/smi.2445

Glare, P., Virik, K., Jones, M., Hudson, M., Eychmuller, S., Simes, J., & Christakis, N. (2003). A systematic review of physicians' survival predictions in terminally ill cancer patients. *BMJ, 327,* 195–198. doi:10.1136/bmj.327.7408.195

Gouin, J.P., Glaser, R., Malarkey, W.B., Beversdorf, D., & Kiecolt-Glaser, J. (2012). Chronic stress, daily stressors, and circulating inflammatory markers. *Health Psychology, 31,* 264–268. doi:10.1037/a0025536

Gravel, K., Légaré, F., & Graham, I.D. (2006). Barriers and facilitators to implementing shared decision-making in clinical practice: A systematic review of health professionals' perceptions. *Implementation Science, 1*, 16. doi:10.1186/1748-5908-1-16

Gurmankin, A.D., Baron, J., Hershey, J.C., & Ubel, P.A. (2002). The role of physicians' recommendations in medical treatment decisions. *Medical Decision Making, 22*, 262–271. doi:10.1177/0272989X0202200314

Hajizadeh, N., Figueroa, R., Uhler, L., Chiou, E., Perchonok, J., & Montague, E. (2013). Identifying design considerations for a shared decision aid for use at the point of outpatient clinical care. *Journal of Participatory Medicine, 5*, E1–E4.

Hall, J.D., Boyd, J.C., Lippert, M.C., & Theodorescu, D. (2003). Why patients choose prostatectomy or brachytherapy for localized prostate cancer: Results of a descriptive survey. *Urology, 61*, 402–407. doi:10.1016/S0090-4295(02)02162-3

Hamilton, J.B., & Sandelowski, M. (2004). Types of social support in African Americans with cancer. *Oncology Nursing Forum, 31*, 792–800. doi:10.1188/04.ONF.792-800

Hardee, J.T., Platt, F.W., & Kasper, I.K. (2005). Discussing health care costs with patients: An opportunity for empathic communication. *Journal of General Internal Medicine, 20*, 666–669. doi:10.1111/j.1525-1497.2005.0125.x

Himmelstein, D.U., Warren, E., Thorne, D., & Woolhandler, S. (2005, February). Market watch: Illness and injury as contributors to bankruptcy. *Health Affairs, W5*, 63–73. doi:10.1377/hlthaff.w5.63

Institute of Medicine. (2001). *Crossing the quality chasm: A new health system for the 21st century*. Washington, DC: National Academies Press.

Jangland, E., Gunningberg, L., & Carlsson, M. (2009). Patients' and relatives' complaints about encounters and communication in health care: Evidence for quality improvement. *Patient Education and Counseling, 75*, 199–204. doi:10.1016/j.pec.2008.10.007

Johnson, R., Roter, D., Powe, N.R., & Cooper, L.A. (2004). Patient race/ethnicity and quality of patient–physician communication during medical visits. *American Journal of Public Health, 94*, 2084–2090. doi:10.2105/AJPH.94.12.2084

Jones, R.A., Steeves, R., Ropka, M.E., & Hollen, P. (2013). Capturing treatment decision making among patients with solid tumors and their caregivers [Online exclusive]. *Oncology Nursing Forum, 40*, E24–E31. doi:10.1188/13.ONF.E24-E31

Jones, R.A., Steeves, R., & Williams, I. (2009). How African American men decide whether or not to get prostate cancer screening. *Cancer Nursing, 32*, 166–172. doi:10.1097/NCC.0b013e3181982c6e

Jones, R.A., Steeves, R., & Williams, I. (2010). Family and friend interactions among African-American men deciding whether to have a prostate cancer screening. *Urologic Nursing, 30*, 189–194. Retrieved from http://www.ncbi.nlm.nih.gov/pmc/articles/PMC3616189

Jones, R.A., Wenzel, J., Hinton, I., Cary, M., Jones, N.R., Krumm, S., & Ford, J.G. (2011). Exploring cancer support needs for older African-American men with prostate cancer. *Supportive Care in Cancer, 19*, 1411–1419. doi:10.1007/s00520-010-0967-x

Keirns, C.C., & Goold, S.D. (2009). Patient-centered care and preference-sensitive decision making. *JAMA, 302*, 1805–1806. doi:10.1001/jama.2009.1550

Kilbridge, K.L., Fraser, G., Krahn, M., Nelson, E.M., Conaway, M., Bashore, R., … Connors, A.F. (2009). Lack of comprehension of common prostate cancer terms in an underserved population. *Journal of Clinical Oncology, 27*, 2015–2021. doi:10.1200/JCO.2008.17.3468

Kim, P. (2007). Cost of cancer care: The patient perspective. *Journal of Clinical Oncology, 25*, 228–232. doi:10.1200/JCO.2006.07.9111

Kutner, M., Greenberg, E., Jin, Y., & Paulsen, C. (2006). *The health literacy of America's adults: Results from the 2003 National Assessment of Adult Literacy* (No. NCES 2006483). Washington, DC: U.S. Department of Education National Center for Education Statistics.

Langa, K.M., Fendrick, A.M., Chernew, M.E., Kabeto, M.U., Paisley, K.L., & Hayman, J.A. (2004). Out-of-pocket health-care expenditures among older Americans with cancer. *Value in Health, 7*, 186–194. doi:10.1111/j.1524-4733.2004.72334.x

Légaré, F., Ratté, S., Stacey, D., Kryworuchko, J., Gravel, K., Graham, I.D., & Turcotte, S. (2010). Interventions for improving the adoption of shared decision making by healthcare professionals. *Cochrane Database of Systematic Reviews, 2010*(5). doi:10.1002/14651858.CD006732.pub2

Liebertz, C., & Fox, P. (2006). Ketoconazole as a secondary hormonal intervention in advanced prostate cancer. *Clinical Journal of Oncology Nursing, 10,* 361–366. doi:10.1188/06.CJON.361-366

Little, M., & Sayers, E.J. (2004). While there's life . . . Hope and the experience of cancer. *Social Science and Medicine, 59,* 1329–1337. doi:10.1016/j.socscimed.2004.01.014

McLennon, S.M., Uhrich, M., Lasiter, S., Chamness, A.R., & Helft, P.R. (2013). Oncology nurses' narratives about ethical dilemmas and prognosis-related communication in advanced cancer patients. *Cancer Nursing, 36,* 114–121. doi:10.1097/NCC.0b013e31825f4dc8

McWilliams, J.M. (2009). Health consequences of uninsurance among adults in the United States: Recent evidence and implications. *Milbank Quarterly, 87,* 443–494. doi:10.1111/j.1468-0009.2009.00564.x

McWilliams, J.M., Meara, E., Zaslavsky, A.M., & Ayanian, J.Z. (2007). Health of previously uninsured adults after acquiring Medicare coverage. *JAMA, 298,* 2886–2894. doi:10.1001/jama.298.24.2886

Meropol, N.J., Schrag, D., Smith, T.J., Mulvey, T.M., Langdon, R.M., Jr., Blum, D., ... Schnipper, L.E. (2009). American Society of Clinical Oncology guidance statement: The cost of cancer care. *Journal of Clinical Oncology, 27,* 3868–3874. doi:10.1200/JCO.2009.23.1183

Musa, D., Schulz, R., Harris, R., Silverman, M., & Thomas, S.B. (2009). Trust in the health care system and the use of preventive health services by older black and white adults. *American Journal of Public Health, 99,* 1293–1299. doi:10.2105/AJPH.2007.123927

National Hospice and Palliative Care Organization. (2015). *NHPCO facts and figures: Hospice care in America* (2015 ed.). Retrieved from http://www.nhpco.org/sites/default/files/public/Statistics_Research/2015_Facts_Figures.pdf

National Institute on Aging. (2011). *Global health and aging* (NIH Publication No. 11-7737). Retrieved from http://www.who.int/ageing/publications/global_health.pdf

Neumann, P.J., Palmer, J.A., Nadler, E., Fang, C., & Ubel, P. (2010). Cancer therapy costs influence treatment: A national survey of oncologists. *Health Affairs, 29,* 196–202. doi:10.1377/hlthaff.2009.0077

O'Connor, A.M., Wennberg, J.E., Légaré, F., Llewellyn-Thomas, H.A., Moulton, B.W., Sepucha, K.R., ... King, J.S. (2007). Toward the 'tipping point': Decision aids and informed patient choice. *Health Affairs, 26,* 716–725. doi:10.1377/hlthaff.26.3.716

Pavlish, C., Brown-Saltzman, K., Hersh, M., Shirk, M., & Nudelman, O. (2011). Early indicators and risk factors for ethical issues in clinical practice. *Journal of Nursing Scholarship, 43,* 13–21. doi:10.1111/j.1547-5069.2010.01380.x

Peek, M.E., Odoms-Young, A., Quinn, M.T., Gorawara-Bhat, R., Wilson, S.C., & Chin, M.H. (2010). Race and shared decision-making: Perspectives of African-Americans with diabetes. *Social Science and Medicine, 71,* 1–9. doi:10.1016/j.socscimed.2010.03.014

Power, T.E., Swartzman, L.C., & Robinson, J.W. (2011). Cognitive-emotional decision making (CEDM): A framework of patient medical decision making. *Patient Education and Counseling, 83,* 163–169. doi:10.1016/j.pec.2010.05.021

Ramfelt, E., & Lützén, K. (2005). Patients with cancer: Their approaches to participation in treatment plan decisions. *Nursing Ethics, 12,* 143–155. doi:10.1191/0969733005ne771oa

Schapira, L. (2008). Communication: What do patients want and need? *Journal of Oncology Practice, 4,* 249–253. doi:10.1200/JOP.0856501

Scheier, D.B. (2009). Barriers to health care for people with hearing loss: A review of the literature. *Journal of the New York State Nurses Association, 40*(1), 4–10.

Schenker, Y., Fernandez, A., Sudore, R., & Schillinger, D. (2011). Interventions to improve patient comprehension in informed consent for medical and surgical procedures: A systematic review. *Medical Decision Making, 31,* 151–173. doi:10.1177/0272989X10364247

Schrag, D., & Hanger, M. (2007). Medical oncologists' views on communicating with patients about chemotherapy costs: A pilot survey. *Journal of Clinical Oncology, 25,* 233–237. doi:10.1200/JCO.2006.09.2437

Seccareccia, D. (2010). Cancer-related hypercalcemia. *Canadian Family Physician, 56,* 244–246.

Skinner, C.S., Schildkraut, J.M., Berry, D., Calingaert, B., Marcom, P.K., Sugarman, J., … Rimer, B.K. (2004). Pre-counseling education materials for *BRCA* testing: Does tailoring make a difference? *Genetic Testing, 6,* 93–105. doi:10.1089/10906570260199348

Smith, M., Flamm, A., & Pentz, R. (2009). Ethical and legal issues in the care of cancer patient. In S. Yeung, C. Escalante, & R. Gagel (Eds.), *Medical care of cancer patients* (pp. 43–52). Shelton, CT: People's Medical Publishing House/BC Decker.

Stacey, D., Légaré, F., Col, N.F., Bennett, C.L., Barry, M.J., Eden, K.B., … Wu, J.H.C. (2014). Decision aids for people facing health treatment or screening decisions. *Cochrane Database of Systematic Reviews, 2014*(1). doi:10.1002/14651858.CD001431.pub4

Temel, J.S., Greer, J.A., Muzikansky, A., Gallagher, E.R., Admane, S., Jackson, V.A., … Lynch, T.J. (2010). Early palliative care for patients with metastatic non-small-cell lung cancer. *New England Journal of Medicine, 363,* 733–742. doi:10.1056/NEJMoa1000678

Teunissen, S.C., de Graeff, A., Voest, E.E., & de Haes, J.C. (2007). Are anxiety and depressed mood related to physical symptom burden? A study in hospitalized advanced cancer patients. *Palliative Medicine, 21,* 341–346. doi:10.1177/0269216307079067

Thekkumpurath, P., Venkateswaran, C., Kumar, M., Newsham, A., & Bennett, M.I. (2009). Screening for psychological distress in palliative care: Performance of touch screen questionnaires compared with semistructured psychiatric interview. *Journal of Pain and Symptom Management, 38,* 597–605. doi:10.1016/j.jpainsymman.2009.01.004

Thomas, W.P., & Collier, V.P. (2009). *English learners in North Carolina, 2009: Executive summary prepared for the North Carolina Department of Public Instruction.* Retrieved from http://esl.ncwiseowl.org/UserFiles/Servers/Server_4502383/File/NC_ELL_Study_Yr1_ExecSummary.pdf

Thorne, S.E., Bultz, B.D., & Baile, W.F. (2005). Is there a cost to poor communication in cancer care? A critical review of the literature. *Psycho-Oncology, 14,* 875–884. doi:10.1002/pon.947

Ulrich, C.M., Taylor, C., Soeken, K., O'Donnell, P., Farrar, A., Danis, M., & Grady, C. (2010). Everyday ethics: Ethical issues and stress in nursing practice. *Journal of Advanced Nursing, 66,* 2510–2519. doi:10.1111/j.1365-2648.2010.05425.x

Viale, P.H., & Yamamoto, D.S. (2008). Cardiovascular toxicity associated with cancer treatment. *Clinical Journal of Oncology Nursing, 12,* 627–638. doi:10.1188/08.CJON.627-638

Wenzel, J., Jones, R., Klimmek, R., Szanton, S., & Krumm, S. (2012). Exploring the role of community health workers in providing cancer navigation: Perceptions of African American older adults [Online exclusive]. *Oncology Nursing Forum, 39,* E288–E298. doi:10.1188/12.ONF.E288-E298

Workman, M.L. (2013). Care of patients with cancer. In D.D. Ignatavicius & M.L. Workman (Eds.), *Medical-surgical nursing: Patient-centered collaborative care* (7th ed., pp. 408–432). St. Louis, MO: Elsevier Saunders.

CHAPTER 4

Palliative and End-of-Life Care

Samuel G. Robbins, DNP, MTS, ANP-BC, ACHPN

Introduction

Both palliative and end-of-life care encompass distinct yet interwoven realms within nursing. Palliative care often is equated with end-of-life care, which is typically provided by hospice. Both providers and the general public commonly confuse the two types of care, partly because the broader palliative care philosophy evolved directly from the hospice model of care (Dahlin & Mazanec, 2011). In addition, nurses and physicians often make no meaningful distinction between palliative care and hospice (Parikh, Kirch, Smith, & Temel, 2013). A recent study found that more than 70% of the general public were unable to accurately define palliative care; however, when provided with a definition, 90% indicated that patients with serious illnesses should have access to this type of care (Center to Advance Palliative Care [CAPC], 2011).

In the past century, modern medicine has radically altered the trajectory of dying. Before this time, medicine was largely incapable of reversing disease and curbing mortality. Intravenous hydration and antibiotic therapy, for instance, did not come into widespread use until the 1950s. Prior to the 20th century, patients who acquired pneumonia would typically either recover promptly or die, and medical interventions were generally palliative at best (Porter, 1997). Today, the dying process typically occurs gradually and to the frail elderly rather than swiftly and to the previously healthy. According to Singleton (2014), 90% of people will experience steady declines in health as a result of multiple progressive illnesses. Medical treatments can prevent death for years or even decades, fostering the appealing illusion that mortality is optional (Kass, 2004). In this fundamentally new cultural context, misunderstandings cloud how palliative care and hospice are interrelated and how they can best be used during a patient's illness and at the end of life.

Although the immense progress made in medicine should be celebrated, its successes have led to a dramatic increase in the number of patients living with serious, life-threatening illnesses. These patient populations are diverse and include all major categories of disease, for example,
• Trauma survivors living with chronic and life-threatening injuries
• Neonates, children, adolescents, and adults who were born with conditions or disabilities that render them dependent on life support or caregivers to maintain health or perform activities of daily living
• Individuals with acute illnesses that are partially reversible but lead to diminished quality of life as a result of burdensome treatment
• Individuals who experience chronic, progressive diseases, including malignancies, advanced lung or heart disease, stroke, renal failure, neurodegenerative disorders, frailty, and dementias
• Terminally ill patients with end-stage diseases for whom stable recovery is no longer achievable and palliative care is the primary emphasis of caregiving interventions
• Socially marginalized and impoverished populations that lack access to healthcare resources (e.g., homeless individuals, individuals with mental illness, immigrants, veterans, prisoners) (National Consensus Project for Quality Palliative Care [NCP], 2013).

Of the six aforementioned categories, only one is specifically devoted to those who are terminally ill and therefore potentially eligible for hospice care. From this broad standpoint, many patients with complex clinical problems who might benefit from specialized palliative care have lengthy prognoses.

This chapter provides an overview of basic concepts and definitions, as well as a discussion of some of the common ethical dilemmas encountered by nurses in palliative and hospice care. In addition, major implications for nursing practice are reviewed, and a case study describes one of the more challenging ethical situations that can occur in these settings.

Concepts and Components of Palliative Care

As might be expected in an emerging specialty like palliative care, definitions vary and are somewhat disputed. The following definition is derived from consumer research and appears to be consistently useful for patients and their families.

> Palliative care is specialized medical care for people with serious illnesses. This type of care is focused on providing patients with relief from the symptoms, pain, and stress of a serious illness—whatever the diagnosis. The goal is to improve quality of

life for both the patient and the family. Palliative care is provided by a team of doctors, nurses, and other specialists who work with a patient's other doctors to provide an extra layer of support. Palliative care is appropriate at any age and at any stage in a serious illness, and can be provided together with curative treatment. (CAPC, 2011, p. 7)

In this definition, palliative care is described as a specialty service that is added to existing services. Astute observers have countered this description by suggesting that primary care clinicians provide the majority of palliative care as a routine part of standard care (von Gunten, 2002).

The World Health Organization (WHO) defines *palliative care* as "an approach that improves the quality of life of patients and their families facing the problem[s] associated with life-threatening illness, through the prevention and relief of suffering by means of early identification and impeccable assessment and treatment of pain and other problems, physical, psychosocial, and spiritual" (WHO, 2015, para. 1).

Palliative care
- Provides relief from pain and other distressing symptoms
- Affirms life and regards dying as a normal process
- Intends neither to hasten nor postpone death
- Integrates the psychological and spiritual aspects of patient care
- Offers a support system to help patients live as actively as possible until death and to help family members cope during the patient's illness and in their own bereavement
- Uses a team approach to address the needs of patients and their families, including bereavement counseling if indicated
- Enhances quality of life and may also positively influence the course of the patient's illness
- Is applicable early in the course of illness and in conjunction with other therapies that are intended to prolong life, such as chemotherapy or radiation therapy, and includes those investigations needed to better understand and manage distressing clinical complications. (WHO, 2015, para. 2)

According to the National Hospice and Palliative Care Organization (NHPCO), "Palliative care is patient and family-centered care that optimizes quality of life by anticipating, preventing, and treating suffering. Palliative care throughout the continuum of illness involves addressing physical, intellectual, emotional, social, and spiritual needs and to facilitate patient autonomy, access to information, and choice" (NHPCO, n.d.). NHPCO (n.d.) cites the following as characteristics of palliative care philosophy and delivery.
- Care is provided and services are coordinated by an interdisciplinary team.
- Patients, families, and palliative and non-palliative healthcare providers collaborate and communicate about care needs.

- Services are available concurrently with or independent of curative or life-prolonging care.
- Patient and family hopes for peace and dignity are supported throughout the course of illness, during the dying process, and after death.

Many major professional medical associations endorse this broad definition. Prominent organizations emphasize that the majority of palliative care should be provided by the primary care team involved with the patient and not by palliative care specialists (Holloway et al., 2014). Many experts further argue that primary care providers should provide the majority of palliative care because it is a core component of quality care. Furthermore, there are simply too few palliative care specialists to meet the demand for patients' palliative care needs (Meier, 2011).

The conceptual aspiration behind each of these definitions is that the care continuum reflects serious illnesses experienced by patients. Figure 4-1 presents an idealized spectrum of how palliative care can be integrated with disease-modifying treatments for patients with cancer.

Narrower definitions, such as WHO's, emphasize a close link between palliative and end-of-life care. Broader definitions of palliative care, however, suggest that it can exist separately from end-of-life care. Understandably, these varying definitions leave many people confused about what palliative care is and is not. Part of the confusion stems from a tacit belief that mortality is a medical problem with a medical solution. As Dr. Ira Byock and other palliative care advocates argue, dying is not fundamentally a medical problem but rather a part of the human condition that requires a range of responses beyond the scope of clinical practice and science (Byock, 2006). Thus, medical approaches are incapable of effectively addressing the existential questions that people confront when faced with mortality. Even so, this review of major definitions of palliative care demon-

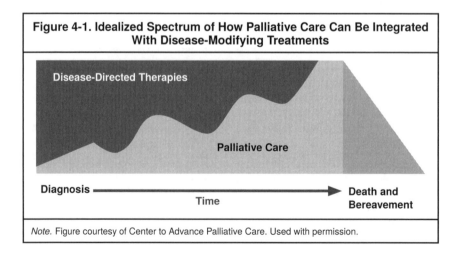

Figure 4-1. Idealized Spectrum of How Palliative Care Can Be Integrated With Disease-Modifying Treatments

Disease-Directed Therapies

Palliative Care

Diagnosis ⟶ Death and Bereavement

Time

Note. Figure courtesy of Center to Advance Palliative Care. Used with permission.

strates common themes emphasizing a holistic philosophy of care that is aimed at improving the quality of life for patients at different stages of disease.

Recently, interdisciplinary consultation teams have begun to provide palliative care in acute care hospitals. These services have increased steadily in larger hospitals over the past 15 years. Today, most hospitals with more than 50 beds have dedicated palliative care staff working to improve care for both dying patients and patients with end-stage illnesses (see Figure 4-2). Expert consensus argues that these consultation teams should be invited to assist patients and families from diagnosis onward; however, palliative care specialists often are not called into the clinical picture until a patient's death is relatively imminent (Andrews & Seymour, 2011). A recent study found that nearly 50% of oncologists avoid consulting palliative care out of concern for potentially alarming patients and families (Smith, C.B., et al., 2012).

Confusion persists among hospital staff about the role of palliative care teams. Because attending physicians often do not consult patients about palliative care until just before the dying process, the presumption is that palliative care occurs only when patients are dying and in urgent need of transition to hospice (Sleeman & Collis, 2013). The popular perception that hospice care is reserved for only

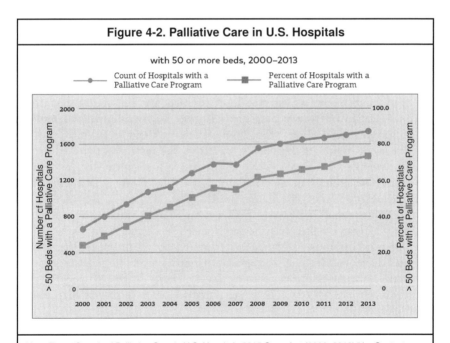

Figure 4-2. Palliative Care in U.S. Hospitals

with 50 or more beds, 2000–2013

Count of Hospitals with a Palliative Care Program

Percent of Hospitals with a Palliative Care Program

Note. From "Growth of Palliative Care in U.S. Hospitals 2015 Snapshot (2000–2013)," by Center to Advance Palliative Care and The National Palliative Care Registry™, 2015. Retrieved from https://www.capc.org/media/filer_public/c5/af/c5afb02e-5e12-47f0-954a-ee23e55ea632/capc_growth_snapshot_2015.pdf. Copyright 2015 by Center to Advance Palliative Care. Reprinted with permission.

those patients who are at the brink of death perpetuates ill-timed end-of-life care, as evidenced by the growing problem of short hospice length of stay (Institute of Medicine [IOM], 2014).

Although community-based outpatient models of delivering non-hospice palliative care have begun to emerge, access remains limited. Developing models for delivering outpatient palliative care promise to benefit patients, families, clinicians, and the healthcare system. Evidence suggests that outpatient palliative care can improve patient satisfaction, symptom management, quality of life, and even survival for some patients with lung cancer (Rabow et al., 2013). Based on the benefits seen in patients with cancer, outpatient integration of palliative care has potential relevance for many patient populations that are burdened by distressing symptoms. Data from randomized controlled trials demonstrating the benefits of palliative care in patients with metastatic cancer who also received standard oncology care have only recently become available (Temel et al., 2010). The vision of outpatient palliative care integration with standard care for patients with metastatic cancer has been embraced by the American Society of Clinical Oncology (Smith, T.J., et al., 2012).

The most well-established form of palliative care is hospice. It is reserved for patients whose prognosis appears to be six months or less and who choose to forgo some interventions for their terminal diagnosis. Since 1982, Medicare has provided funding for hospice services. Most private insurances have followed Medicare's lead by also paying for hospice services. Hospice does not reduce life expectancy and appears to be associated with longer survival for certain disease trajectories (Bruera & Yennurajalingam, 2011). While the use of hospice care has increased, most patients' enrollment in hospice is for less than three weeks, which may limit the benefits they might gain from these services. In fact, over the past two decades, the overall median length of stay in hospice has declined 40%, from 29 days to about 17 (Lynn, Schuster, Wilkinson, & Simon, 2007; NHPCO, 2015). The reasons for short hospice stays are complex, but experts consistently report that part of the problem is related to deficient communication among patients, families, and physicians (Teno, Casarett, Spence, & Connor, 2012).

Today, approximately 45% of U.S. citizens die while in hospice care, a percentage that has nearly doubled over the past decade (Teno et al., 2013). In 2014, just over one-third of hospice patients had a terminal cancer diagnosis; non-cancer terminal diagnoses, such as dementia, congestive heart failure, and chronic obstructive pulmonary disease, account for a majority of hospice beneficiaries. Patients in hospice are cared for by an interdisciplinary team (see Figure 4-3) (NHPCO, 2015).

In hospice care, patients receive intermittent nursing care and 24-hour availability for acute needs. Hospice teams' core responsibilities are to manage patients' symptoms and address the emotional, psychosocial, and spiritual aspects of dying. Drugs, medical supplies, and equipment are provided as well. A range of other services, such as counseling and bereavement, are offered in an effort to provide

Figure 4-3. Interdisciplinary Hospice Caregivers

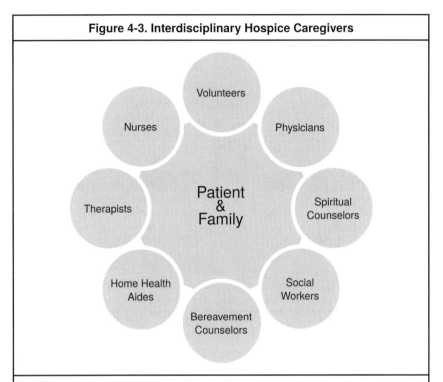

Note. From *NHPCO's Facts and Figures: Hospice Care in America* (2015 ed., p. 3), by National Hospice and Palliative Care Organization, 2015. Retrieved from http://www.nhpco.org/sites/default/files/public/Statistics_Research/2015_Facts_Figures.pdf. Copyright 2015 by National Hospice and Palliative Care Organization. Reprinted with permission.

patient-centered and family-oriented care. The vast majority of patients in hospice care receive services where they live, with approximately one-quarter of beneficiaries using inpatient hospice care for part or all of their stay (NHPCO, 2015). Inpatient hospice is typically reserved for those patients suffering acute symptoms that cannot feasibly be managed at a less resource-intensive level of care.

Dame Cicely Saunders is considered the founder of the modern hospice movement. Her concept of "total pain" articulates the ambition of palliative care to address human suffering in its complexity. As a patient's health declines, pain occurs on different levels. Physical pain is just one aspect of the suffering normally experienced by patients with serious illnesses (see Figure 4-4).

As patients and families transition from non-hospice modes of palliation into formal end-of-life and hospice care, the dynamics of total pain often come into the foreground and may require specialty level palliative care to effectively improve symptoms of distress. The purpose of interdisciplinary palliative care teams is to ensure access to the expertise necessary to alleviate pain in its various dimensions.

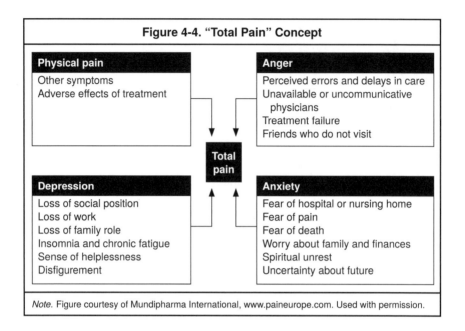

Figure 4-4. "Total Pain" Concept

Physical pain
Other symptoms
Adverse effects of treatment

Anger
Perceived errors and delays in care
Unavailable or uncommunicative
  physicians
Treatment failure
Friends who do not visit

Total pain

Depression
Loss of social position
Loss of work
Loss of family role
Insomnia and chronic fatigue
Sense of helplessness
Disfigurement

Anxiety
Fear of hospital or nursing home
Fear of pain
Fear of death
Worry about family and finances
Spiritual unrest
Uncertainty about future

Note. Figure courtesy of Mundipharma International, www.paineurope.com. Used with permission.

Common Ethical Dilemmas in Palliative Care

Ethical issues routinely arise in palliative care, particularly in end-of-life scenarios. Five of the most common problems relevant to oncology nursing are briefly reviewed here. They involve deficient communication, provision of non-beneficial care, disregard for patient autonomy, issues with symptom management and opioid use, and questions about decision making (Cheon, Coyle, Wiegand, & Welsh, 2015).

Deficient communication among healthcare providers can adversely affect patient care. Nurses, in particular, may experience moral distress when a patient and family appear to lack the information necessary to make prudent decisions in complex circumstances (Ferrell, 2006). This distress can be especially acute when inadequate intraprofessional communication among physicians leads to patients receiving mixed or incomplete messages; with five or more physicians seeing a typical palliative care patient during a single acute care hospitalization, this confusion is unsurprising. A prime example of this communication deficiency is evidenced by a recent study showing that a clear majority of patients with terminal cancer believe that their chemotherapy treatments are curative and not merely palliative (Weeks et al., 2012). The foundation of palliative care ethics relies on providers working to enhance communication so patients can make informed decisions. When armed with a coherent understanding of clinical realities, patients and families overwhelmingly tend to make rational decisions. Earlier end-of-life discussions have been shown to curtail the use of aggressive interventions at the end of life and increase the use of hospice within terminal cancer patient populations (Mack et al., 2012; Obermeyer et al., 2014).

Providers sometimes offer nonbeneficial treatments either because they fail to recognize that a patient is dying or because a patient or family insists on it. In other instances, both healthcare professionals and families are complicit in continuing interventions that are more burdensome than beneficial to the patient. In these scenarios, the purpose of palliative care is to improve communication and help providers and families avoid subjecting patients to ineffective interventions that may prolong suffering. Families and patients often have unrealistic expectations of medicine's capacity to reverse or cure disease processes (Nelson & Hope, 2012). Physicians are sometimes unwilling or unable to communicate directly that a patient is dying. In other instances, physicians fear legal reprisal and acquiesce to perceived patient or family demands. Patients or families commonly request nonbeneficial interventions, such as cardiopulmonary resuscitation, because they lack valid information about the actual risks and benefits of procedures (Weissman, 2001).

Patient autonomy may be threatened when a family requests that information about medical decisions be withheld from the patient. An example of this is when a family requests to contradict a patient's clear advance directive. Another example is when a family decides to transfer the patient to hospice care but insists that hospital staff not mention the word *hospice* in the presence of the patient. These requests typically arise from fear that doing so will diminish the patient's capacity for hope. Eliciting the family's reason for wishing to conceal information from the patient is typically the first step in resolving the conflict. Inviting patients to discuss specific care goals and evaluating these for congruence with hospice services is typically the second step in addressing requests for concealing hospice involvement from patients.

Palliative care specialists are frequently asked to mediate conflicts concerning patient autonomy in end-of-life contexts. It is often unclear, particularly in acute care settings, if patients genuinely have decision-making capacity and can exercise their autonomy. Clinicians also may disagree as to whether a patient retains the ability to choose among plans of care. Nurses can advocate for patient-centered care in these instances by clearly communicating their assessments about patient capacity or specifics about patient wishes to all members of the clinical team as well as to the appropriate family members. In cases where it is clear that a patient lacks capacity to participate meaningfully in complex medical decisions, surrogate decision makers will sometimes make choices incongruent with what nurses believe is beneficial. In these instances, ethical conflicts around decision making arise, and nurses hold a professional duty to advocate for the patient. Palliative care specialists are commonly called upon in these situations to help establish beneficial goals of care by providing emotional and clinical support to anxious families as well as to professional caregivers experiencing moral distress.

As patients and families navigate end-of-life scenarios, advance directives can be useful tools for protecting patients from getting medical interventions that are inconsistent with their preferences (Silveira, Wiitala, & Piette, 2014). Although these documents most often do not provide ready-made answers to clinical situations, they can provide a helpful means of guiding patients, families, and caregivers through difficult medical decision making. Emotionally taxing conversations related to questions surrounding code status and different modes of artificial life support can be addressed by living wills. Furthermore, specialized forms called Physician Orders for Life-Sustaining Treatment (POLST), or Physician Orders for Scope of Treatment (POST), translate patient preferences into medical orders that move with the patient across settings (National POLST Paradigm, 2015). These forms appear to increase the likelihood that patients will receive medical treatment consistent with their wishes. A recent review based on records from Oregon showed that patients who completed POLST forms indicating they wanted only comfort measures stood better than a 93% chance of avoiding death in a hospital. Conversely, patients whose forms indicated a desire for no limitations on medical interventions were nearly 10 times more likely to die in a hospital (Fromme, Zive, Schmidt, Cook, & Tolle, 2014).

Nurses often face ethical dilemmas related to symptom management, particularly in the case of opioid administration. Because of tolerance to opioids and other contributing symptoms, some patients with chronic pain require higher and higher doses of opioids as their pain increases in severity, and nurses may become uncomfortable administering unusually high doses of narcotics. Employing Cicely Saunders' concept of "total pain," nurses can invite patients to explore the dynamics of their suffering, often revealing sources of pain that are predominantly psychosocial or spiritual in nature. In palliative and end-of-life scenarios, nurses frequently report discomfort with expectations to administer doses of analgesics they worry may hasten death through overmedication, though in actuality this is unlikely (Barnett, Mulvenon, Dalrymple, & Connelly, 2010; Hallenbeck, 2012). At other times, nurses report frustration with physicians' apparent unwillingness to prescribe opioids at doses sufficient to alleviate severe pain (Long et al., 2010). Nurses also report distress during cases of palliative sedation where concerns about hastening death enter the clinical foreground (Hospice and Palliative Nurses Association [HPNA], 2011). In navigating these difficult scenarios, nurses can find robust professional support from the American Nurses Association's (ANA's) position statement on end-of-life care (2010) and *Code of Ethics for Nurses With Interpretive Statements* (2015), as well as the HPNA position statement (2011).

Implications for Nursing Practice

According to Provision 1 of ANA's *Code of Ethics for Nurses*, nurses are duty-bound to advocate specifically for dying patients (ANA, 2015). Moreover, patients need to live with as much well-being—physically, psychologically, and spiritually—as possible, and this imperative is integrated throughout the *Code of Ethics for Nurses* and is fundamental to nursing practice. Nurses might consider themselves palliative care advocates. In light of a growing body of evidence, early palliative care interventions—initiated months or years before a patient's death—have the power to foster conditions conducive to quality end-of-life care. Through the use of tools such as advance care planning; thoughtful conversations among providers, patients, and families; and symptom management, death can be made far less difficult than it too often is (IOM, 2014).

Nurses can effectively advocate for palliative care by educating colleagues about the interdisciplinary approach of specialty level palliative care. When colleagues reduce palliative care to end-of-life or hospice care, nurses can clarify that serious illness at any stage affects patients and families physically, emotionally, socially, and spiritually; therefore, earlier palliative care referral may be beneficial. The Oncology Nursing Society's (2014) position statement on palliative care advocates palliative care commencing at diagnosis. Nurses also can tactfully refer colleagues to the American Society of Clinical Oncology guidelines, which advocate for earlier integration of palliative care for patients with cancer who have a high symptom burden or metastatic disease (Smith, T.J., et al., 2012). Data suggest that as many as 4 in 10 patients with cancer receive suboptimal pain management, indicating a considerable need for the intensified symptom management that quality palliative medicine provides (Smith, C.B., et al., 2012). Nurses also can point out that the basic goal of palliative care is to improve quality of life for patients and families throughout any serious disease process. Patients with oxygen-dependent chronic obstructive pulmonary disease, advanced congestive heart failure, end-stage renal disease, or progressive neurodegenerative diseases typically experience severe symptoms that palliative care expertise may be able to effectively ameliorate. Moreover, patients living with cancer or any serious illness experience suffering beyond physical pain (Mehta & Chan, 2008). Addressing the psychosocial and spiritual distress associated with serious illness is fundamental to both palliative care interventions and nursing advocacy (NCP, 2013).

Specialty level palliative care can enhance and deepen communication among the primary care team, patient, and family. Serious and especially progressive life-limiting illnesses produce profound physical and psychological suffering. Conversations between physicians and patients about the trajectory of disease progression, end of life, and goals of care have been shown to lead to less aggressive interventions and higher quality of life when patients are dying. When handled competently, these conversations do not cause psychological harm, as is often feared. In fact, when such conversations are avoided, psychological and even physical harm appear more likely outcomes (Wright et al., 2008).

In this context, perhaps the most crucial rule of patient-centered communication is obtaining a patient's or family member's permission to discuss issues related to disease progression and end-of-life care (Back, Arnold, & Tulsky, 2009). Patients and families who wish to opt out of conversations about mortality have a right to decline. For the vast majority of patients who welcome gentle invitations to discuss care preferences as their diseases progress, nurses are uniquely positioned to advocate that these conversations reliably occur between providers and patients (Wenger, Asakura, Fink, & Oman, 2012). Further, nurses can play a unique role in discerning when patients and families with complex needs may benefit from specialty level palliative care team involvement. Effective advocacy requires good communication skills with physicians, patients, and families.

Nearly all patients have higher priorities than quantity of life. By engaging in conversations about goals of care, patients make more beneficial medical choices than they might otherwise. What is dreadful can become tolerable, and medicine can serve patients rather than control the remainder of their lives. Moreover, patients and families report feeling relieved when goals and preferences for end-of-life care achieve expression (Gawande, 2014; Wright et al., 2008). For many, these difficult conversations create opportunities to maximize quality of life as quantity runs short. In the absence of discussions about the benefits of palliative care, the medical system dependably maintains its defaults, providing the most aggressive services available. Ultimately, palliative care aspires to counterbalance medicine's emphasis on survival with a commitment to well-being in the face of serious illness and mortality (Gawande, 2014).

The poor quality of end-of-life care provided by the U.S. healthcare system's default modes of intervention has been repeatedly documented over the past two decades, most recently by the IOM report *Dying in America: Improving Quality and Honoring Individual Preferences Near the End of Life* (IOM, 2014). Although the emergence of palliative care as a specialty has begun to change practice patterns for a minority of patients and families, the larger reality is that until most clinicians integrate core palliative care principles into their practice, patient-centered end-of-life care will remain extraordinary rather than standard. Nurses will play a leading role as healthcare systems incorporate primary palliative care interventions into the care of patients with serious illnesses (Nelson et al., 2011). Perhaps the chief implication for nursing is that primary palliative care education and skills should become fundamental to our professional identity.

Case Study

Joseph Donovan is a 56-year-old married man who is admitted to the hospital in pain crisis with widely metastatic lung cancer. The cancer has invaded his pelvis, and he is no longer able to ambulate without maximum assistance. The prior week, he was working part time at his office job. He is intermittently confused, and it is unclear whether he can be considered decisional given his needs for IV opioids and anxiolytics. His oncologist has offered "salvage" chemotherapy, claiming that it offers a "small" chance of benefiting Mr. Donovan to the point where he might be able to walk again. The bedside nurse privately asks the oncologist to quantify "small" chance, and the oncologist states that there is about a 5% chance that the chemotherapy will provide any benefit to the patient. It is clear that the patient's prognosis is weeks to months under any circumstances.

The oncologist consults the hospital's palliative care team when the patient's young adult children begin openly arguing about whether to pursue purely palliative goals of care and transition to hospice or to begin chemotherapy. When his care team asks him about his treatment preferences, Mr. Donovan says he is uncertain but indicates a willingness to consider both options. The patient's wife voices anger that chemotherapy is being offered. One of the patient's children accuses her mother of "trying to kill" her father by pursuing hospice instead.

Admission documentation names the patient's wife as the healthcare power of attorney. Given the clinical consensus that the patient cannot be considered decisional, plans are made to pursue hospice care at the wife's request. The following day, the patient's children claim to have healthcare power of attorney and produce a document that was signed the previous day by the patient. The patient is confused, and one of the children angrily forbids all clinical staff from speaking with his father about hospice or his plan of care. An ethics consult is obtained, and the recommendation is to disregard the newly signed form because the patient signed it when he was clearly nondecisional. Meanwhile, the patient's wife informs the team caring for her husband that she has decided to defer medical decision making to her children, fearing the potential damage to her long-term relationship with them.

Discussion

In cases like Mr. Donovan's, how should nurses respond to family conflict? What are the ethical standards that should shape nurses' thinking and actions in similar scenarios? Using ethical principles that are fundamental to palliative care, nurses can respond constructively and compassionately in situations where it can seem as if hostilities will only escalate. Relevant concepts include understanding dying as a meaning-making experience, viewing suffering as a threat to patient and family integrity, and approaching the conflicts as opportunities for families to discover ways of becoming whole again amid the brokenness that terminal disease inflicts (Partington & Kirk, 2015).

In Mr. Donovan's situation, nurses can address the anticipatory grief of family members, assess their understanding of feasible outcomes for Mr. Donovan, and provide updates about Mr. Donovan's condition. Nurses can suggest that family members be present with Mr. Donovan and focus on ways to alleviate his suffering. The palliative care team recommends giving the family a few days to communicate on their own terms rather than challenging them with ultimatums related to the hospital's interest in discharging the patient.

Within a few days, the family and patient arrive at a consensus for inpatient hospice care. The patient spends the last month of his life in hospice. Family conflicts continued but ultimately lead to the restoration of family integrity and palpable gratitude for the palliative care provided. The patient's bereaved family members report benefiting from the interdisciplinary support of the care team, particularly the support provided by the social worker and chaplain. By employing clinical sensitivity to Mr. Donovan's case, nurses were able to assist the patient and family through a profound period of loss that became, in some ways, a healing experience.

Conclusion

Hospice and palliative care are often confused by the general public (Parikh et al., 2013). Hospice is often perceived as brink-of-death care and palliative care as an elective precursor to hospice. Progress has been made toward making end-of-life care more patient centered and family oriented, but improvement appears uneven at best. Recent studies suggest that dying, from the standpoint of symptom burden, has become more difficult (Singer et al., 2015). From a broad historical standpoint, modern palliative care and hospice represent a retrieval of nursing's ancient traditions of providing comfort in the face of dying and its attendant suffering (Sherman, 2011). Palliative care's bold ambitions to provide comprehensive symptom management, as well as emotional, psychosocial, and spiritual support, remains more of an ideal than a reality. As the discussion and definitions reviewed here suggest, palliative care must be strongly interdisciplinary.

Strong evidence suggests that social determinants shape the experience of health and illness to a far greater degree than purely clinical factors (Frieden, 2010). Palliative care is integrated into interdisciplinary teams, acknowledging this public health reality. Further, mortality ultimately is not a medical problem to be solved. Instead, we are pressed to grapple with existential and spiritual questions well beyond the purview of clinical science (Kass, 2004). The modern biomedical model remains largely dismissive of the spiritual domain despite the fact that authentic palliative care is virtually impossible to provide without embracing patients as whole persons (Kearney, 2009). Close consideration of the palliative care definitions reviewed here suggests that the care of the seriously ill requires nurses to respond to patients as body, mind, and spirit. Failing to do so suggests that palliative nursing's commitment to holistic care amounts to little more than hollow rhetoric. Articulating the fundamental differences and similarities between palliative and hospice care is a first step toward advocating for the appropriate use of both types of care.

References

American Nurses Association. (2010). Registered nurses' roles and responsibilities in providing expert care and counseling at the end of life [Position statement]. Retrieved from http://www .nursingworld.org/MainMenuCategories/Policy-Advocacy/Positions-and-Resolutions/ ANAPositionStatements/Position-Statements-Alphabetically/etpain14426.pdf

American Nurses Association. (2015). *Code of ethics for nurses with interpretive statements.* Retrieved from http://www.nursingworld.org/MainMenuCategories/EthicsStandards/Codeof EthicsforNurses

Andrews, N., & Seymour, J. (2011). Factors influencing the referral of non-cancer patients to community specialist palliative care nurses. *International Journal of Palliative Nursing, 17*, 35–41. doi:10.12968/ijpn.2011.17.1.35

Back, A., Arnold, R., & Tulsky, J. (2009). *Mastering communication with seriously ill patients: Balancing honesty with empathy and hope.* New York, NY: Cambridge University Press.

Barnett, M.L., Mulvenon, C.J., Dalrymple, P.A., & Connelly, L.M. (2010). Nurses' knowledge, attitudes, and practice patterns regarding titration of opioid infusions at the end of life. *Journal of Hospice and Palliative Nursing, 12*, 81–88. doi:10.1097/NJH.0b013e3181cf791c

Bruera, E., & Yennurajalingam, S. (Eds.). (2011). *Oxford American handbook of hospice and palliative medicine.* New York, NY: Oxford University Press.

Byock, I. (2006). Where do we go from here? A palliative care perspective. *Critical Care Medicine, 34*, S416–S420. doi:10.1097/01.CCM.0000237345.62823.82

Center to Advance Palliative Care. (2011). *2011 public opinion research on palliative care: A report based on research by public opinion strategies.* Retrieved from https://www.capc.org/media/filer_public/18/ab/18ab708c-f835-4380-921d-fbf729702e36/2011-public-opinion-research-on-palliative-care.pdf

Cheon, J., Coyle, N., Wiegand, D.L., & Welsh, S. (2015). Ethical issues experienced by hospice and palliative nurses. *Journal of Hospice and Palliative Nursing, 17*, 7–13. doi:10.1097/NJH.0000000000000129

Dahlin, C.M., & Mazanec, P. (2011). Building from our past: Celebrating 25 years of clinical practice in hospice and palliative nursing. *Journal of Hospice and Palliative Nursing, 13*, S20–S28. doi:10.1097/NJH.0b013e3182331016

Ferrell, B.R. (2006). Understanding the moral distress of nurses witnessing medically futile care. *Oncology Nursing Forum, 33*, 922–930. doi:10.1188/06.ONF.922-930

Frieden, T.R. (2010). A framework for public health action: The health impact pyramid. *American Journal of Public Health, 100*, 590–595. doi:10.2105/AJPH.2009.185652

Fromme, E.K., Zive, D., Schmidt, T.A., Cook, J.N., & Tolle, S.W. (2014). Association between physician orders for life-sustaining treatment for scope of treatment and in-hospital death in Oregon. *Journal of the American Geriatrics Society, 62*, 1246–1251. doi:10.1111/jgs.12889

Gawande, A. (2014). *Being mortal: Medicine and what matters in the end.* New York, NY: Metropolitan Books.

Hallenbeck, J. (2012). Pathophysiologies of dyspnea explained: Why might opioids relieve dyspnea and not hasten death? *Journal of Palliative Medicine, 15*, 848–853. doi:10.1089/jpm.2011.0167

Holloway, R.G., Arnold, R.M., Creutzfeldt, C.J., Lewis, E.F., Lutz, B.J., McCann, R.M., … Zorowitz, R.D. (2014). AHA/ASA scientific statement: Palliative and end-of-life care in stroke: A statement for healthcare professionals from the American Heart Association/American Stroke Association. Retrieved from http://my.americanheart.org/idc/groups/ahamah-public/@wcm/@sop/@smd/documents/downloadable/ucm_471261.pdf

Hospice and Palliative Nurses Association. (2011). HPNA position statement: Palliative sedation. Retrieved from http://hpna.advancingexpertcare.org/wp-content/uploads/2014/09/Palliative-Sedation-PositionStatement-080311.pdf

Institute of Medicine. (2014). *Dying in America: Improving quality and honoring individual preferences near the end of life.* Retrieved from http://www.nap.edu/catalog/18748/dying-in-america-improving-quality-and-honoring-individual-preferences-near

Kass, L.R. (2004). L'chaim and its limits: Why not immortality? In S.G. Post & R.H. Binstock (Eds.), *The fountain of youth: Cultural, scientific, and ethical perspectives on a biomedical goal* (pp. 304–320). New York, NY: Oxford University Press.

Kearney, M. (2009). *A place of healing: Working with nature and soul at the end of life.* New Orleans, LA: Spring Journal Books.

Long, C.O., Morgan, B.M., Alonzo, T.R., Mitchell, K.M., Bonnell, D.K., & Beardsley, M.E. (2010). Improving pain management in long-term care: The campaign against pain. *Journal of Hospice and Palliative Nursing, 12*, 148–155. doi:10.1097/NJH.0b013e3181d94f1b

Lynn, J., Schuster, J.L., Wilkinson, A.M., & Simon, L.N. (2007). *Improving care for the end of life: A sourcebook for health care managers and clinicians* (2nd ed.). New York, NY: Oxford University Press.

Mack, J.W., Cronin, A., Keating, N.L., Taback, N., Huskamp, H.A., Malin, J.L., ... Weeks, J.C. (2012). Associations between end-of-life discussion characteristics and care received near death: A prospective cohort study. *Journal of Clinical Oncology, 30,* 4387–4395. doi:10.1200/JCO.2012.43.6055

Meier, D.E. (2011). Increased access to palliative care and hospice services: Opportunities to improve value in health care. *Milbank Quarterly, 89,* 343–380. doi:10.1111/j.1468-0009.2011.00632.x

National Consensus Project for Quality Palliative Care. (2013). *Clinical practice guidelines for quality palliative care* (3rd ed.). Retrieved from http://www.nationalconsensusproject.org

National Hospice and Palliative Care Organization. (n.d.). Palliative care. Retrieved from http://www.nhpco.org/palliative-care-4

National Hospice and Palliative Care Organization. (2015). *NHPCO's facts and figures: Hospice care in America* (2015 ed.). Retrieved from http://www.nhpco.org/sites/default/files/public/Statistics_Research/2015_Facts_Figures.pdf

National POLST Paradigm. (2015). What is POLST? Retrieved from http://www.polst.org/about-the-national-polst-paradigm/what-is-polst

Nelson, J.E., Cortez, T.B., Curtis, J.R., Lustbader, D.R., Mosenthal, A.C., Mulkerin, C., ... Puntillo, K.A. (2011). Integrating palliative care in the ICU: The nurse in a leading role. *Journal of Hospice and Palliative Nursing, 13,* 89–94. doi:10.1097/NJH.0b013e318203d9ff

Nelson, J.E., & Hope, A.A. (2012). Integration of palliative care in chronic critical illness management. *Respiratory Care, 57,* 1004–1013. doi:10.4187/respcare.01624

Obermeyer, Z., Makar, M., Abujaber, S., Dominici, F., Block, S., & Cutler, D.M. (2014). Association between the Medicare hospice benefit and health care utilization and costs for patients with poor-prognosis cancer. *JAMA, 312,* 1888–1896. doi:10.1001/jama.2014.14950

Oncology Nursing Society. (2014). Palliative care for people with cancer [Position statement]. Retrieved from https://www.ons.org/advocacy-policy/positions/practice/palliative-care

Parikh, R.B., Kirch, R.A., Smith, T.J., & Temel, J.S. (2013). Early specialty palliative care—Translating data in oncology into practice. *New England Journal of Medicine, 369,* 2347–2351. doi:10.1056/NEJMsb1305469

Partington, E.W., & Kirk, T.W. (2015). Engaging requests for nondisclosure during admission to home hospice care. *Journal of Hospice and Palliative Nursing, 17,* 174–180. doi:10.1097/NJH.0000000000000157

Porter, R. (1997). *The greatest benefit to mankind: A medical history of humanity.* New York, NY: W.W. Norton and Company.

Rabow, M., Kvale, E., Barbour, L., Cassel, J.B., Cohen, S., Jackson, V., ... Weissman, D. (2013). Moving upstream: A review of the evidence of the impact of outpatient palliative care. *Journal of Palliative Medicine, 16,* 1540–1549. doi:10.1089/jpm.2013.0153

Sherman, D.W. (2011). Nursing and palliative care. In G. Hanks, N.I. Cherny, N.A. Christakis, M. Fallon, S. Kaasa, & R.K. Portenoy (Eds.), *Oxford textbook of palliative medicine* (pp. 177–183). New York, NY: Oxford University Press.

Silveira, M.J., Wiitala, W., & Piette, J. (2014). Advance directive completion by elderly Americans: A decade of change. *Journal of the American Geriatrics Society, 62,* 706–710. doi:10.1111/jgs.12736

Singer, A.E., Meeker, D., Teno, J.M., Lynn, J., Lunney, J.R., & Lorenz, K.A. (2015). Symptom trends in the last year of life from 1998 to 2010: A cohort study. *Annals of Internal Medicine, 162,* 175–183. doi:10.7326/M13-1609

Singleton, J.K., DiGregorio, R.V., Green-Hernandez, C., Holzemer, S.P., Faber, E.S., Ferrara, L.R., & Slyer, J.T. (Eds.). (2014). *Primary care: An interprofessional perspective.* New York, NY: Springer.

Sleeman, K.E., & Collis, E. (2013). Caring for a dying patient in hospital. *BMJ, 346,* f2174. doi:10.1136/bmj.f2174

Smith, C.B., Nelson, J.E., Berman, A.R., Powell, C.A., Fleischman, J., Salazar-Schicchi, J., & Wisnivesky, J.P. (2012). Lung cancer physicians' referral practices for palliative care consultation. *Annals of Oncology, 23,* 382–387. doi:10.1093/annonc/mdr345

Smith, T.J., Temin, S., Alesi, E.R., Abernethy, A.P., Balboni, T.A., Basch, E.M., ... Von Roenn, J.H. (2012). American Society of Clinical Oncology provisional clinical opinion: The integration of palliative care into standard oncology care. *Journal of Clinical Oncology, 30*, 880–887. doi:10.1200/JCO.2011.38.5161

Temel, J.S., Greer, J.A., Muzikansky, A., Gallagher, E.R., Admane, S., Jackson, V.A., & Lynch, T.J. (2010). Early palliative care for patients with metastatic non–small-cell lung cancer. *New England Journal of Medicine, 363*, 733–742.

Teno, J.M., Casarett, D., Spence, C., & Connor, S. (2012). It is "too late" or is it? Bereaved family member perceptions of hospice referral when their family member was on hospice for seven days or less. *Journal of Pain and Symptom Management, 43*, 732–738. doi:10.1016/j.jpainsymman.2011.05.012

Teno, J.M., Gozalo, P.L., Bynum, J.P., Leland, N.E., Miller, S.C., Morden, N.E., ... Mor, V. (2013). Change in end-of-life care for Medicare beneficiaries: Site of death, place of care, and health care transitions in 2000, 2005, and 2009. *JAMA, 309*, 470–477. doi:10.1001/jama.2012.207624

von Gunten, C.F. (2002). Secondary and tertiary palliative care in U.S. hospitals. *JAMA, 287*, 875–881. doi:10.1001/jama.287.7.875

Weeks, J.C., Catalano, P.J., Cronin, A., Finkelman, M.D., Mack, J.W., Keating, N.L., & Schrag, D. (2012). Patients' expectations about effects of chemotherapy for advanced cancer. *New England Journal of Medicine, 367*, 1616–1625. doi:10.1056/NEJMoa1204410

Weissman, D.E. (2001). Managing conflicts at the end of life. *Journal of Palliative Medicine, 4*, 1–3. doi:10.1089/109662101300051843

Wenger, B., Asakura, Y., Fink, R.M., & Oman, K.S. (2012). Dissemination of the five wishes advance directive at work. *Journal of Hospice and Palliative Nursing, 14*, 551–558. doi:10.1097/NJH.0b013e31825ebae0

World Health Organization. (2015). WHO definition of palliative care. Retrieved from http://www.who.int/cancer/palliative/definition/en

Wright, A.A., Zhang, B., Ray, A., Mack, J.W., Trice, E., Balboni, T., ... Prigerson, H.G. (2008). Associations between end-of-life discussions, patient mental health, medical care near death, and caregiver bereavement adjustment. *JAMA, 300*, 1665–1673. doi:10.1001/jama.300.14.1665

CHAPTER 5

Patient Advocacy

Jessica Keim-Malpass, PhD, RN

Introduction

Within the past several decades, caring for patients with cancer has become increasingly complex, as monumental technologic and treatment advancements have occurred. At the same time, healthcare systems have grown larger and more difficult to navigate, with the potential for fragmented care delivery systems. Additionally, passage and implementation of the Patient Protection and Affordable Care Act (ACA) has raised questions regarding healthcare reform and the right to equitable healthcare coverage. A passion for working with the oncology population often carries nurses through challenges in practice, service, and research. Patient advocacy is one lens to use when approaching and understanding this intricate and multifactorial undertaking. This chapter will discuss the epistemological and ontological underpinnings of patient advocacy, examine advocacy's action-based application to ethical nursing practice, and introduce theoretical and empirical referents of patient advocacy. Clinical case studies will be used to describe patient advocacy in practice and to discuss the implications for nurses.

Basic Concepts and Definitions

Patient advocacy is a key concept of clinical nursing practice and is fundamental to the application of nursing ethics. Broadly defined, an advocate is one who defends, pleads the cause of, promotes the rights of, or attempts to change systems on behalf of an individual or group (Jezewski, 1993). The word *advocate* originally stems from the Greek word *advokar*, meaning "one who pleads on the behalf of another" (Sutor, 1993). The concept of advocacy also can be interpreted as "one who is summoned to give evidence," and advocacy *actions* often are defined as verbal support or argumentation for a cause (Vaartio & Leino-Kilpi, 2005). The term *advocacy* has appeared in the nursing literature for almost three decades, and much of it involves legitimizing the nurse's role in advocacy on behalf of patients (Mallik, 1997). The difficulty with conceptualizing this term lies in its diversity in its action-based activities. Advocacy is described as a prerequisite to or an outcome of nursing practice in situations involving decision making, moral and ethical reasoning, patient autonomy, or patient empowerment (Snowball, 1996). This chapter will attempt to clarify the concept of patient advocacy; define the concept's attributes, antecedents, and consequences; and develop a conceptual framework of patient advocacy to be used in oncology nursing practice and research.

Historical Significance

Florence Nightingale is considered to be the first example of a nurse serving as a patient advocate as she emphasized measures whereby environmental factors can be manipulated to put patients in the best condition for nature to act upon them (Bu & Jezewski, 2006). From a historical context, advocacy has not always been central to the understanding of the nurse's professional role; for most of nursing's existence, virtues of unquestioning obedience and loyalty to the physician were primary expectations, leaving little room for nurses to work as patient advocates (Hamric, 2000). In the early 1960s, nurse leaders sought to determine how nurses could develop a unique professional identity beyond the "leftover" tasks associated with the physician. The developing role of nurse advocate was seen as integral in expanding a clinical niche within nursing practice (Snowball, 1996).

In the 1970s, a shift toward increased attention on patients' rights occurred as a result of progress in the U.S. legal system and the rise of the consumer movement as an attempt to equalize power between healthcare providers and patients (Annas & Healey, 1974). In the United States, this shift to a consumer movement has been attributed to the general public attaining higher levels of education, an awareness of the powers and dangers of new medical technology, distrust of experts, and the Civil Rights movement (Mallik, 1997). In the 1980s, advocacy took on a social context as it began to be targeted toward vulnerable populations, particularly during the advent of the HIV/AIDS epidemic (Copp, 1986). During this time, the nurse advocate role evolved as being both a resource person and a watchdog, monitoring the clarity of information to protect patients (Snowball, 1996). Today, patient-centered health care is still driving autonomy in decision making as well as ensuring medical safety and quality and the rights of patients and families. Vulnerable groups are still considered within the context of advocacy and are the focus of many advocacy efforts.

Advocacy and Nursing Practice Guidelines

Advocacy first appeared as a practice guideline in 1988 in the United Kingdom's Project 2000 nursing curriculum, with guidelines stating that advocacy is a condition of contemporary nursing practice (Baldwin, 2003). Today, the International Council of Nurses' (ICN's) *Code of Ethics for Nurses* requires that nurses advocate for and protect the health, well-being, safety, values, and rights of all patients in the healthcare system (ICN, 2012). Hamric (2000) suggested that although advocacy is a part of today's theoretical-based curricula in nursing education, a disconnect still exists in the concept being a central component of clinical practice. It is important to consider how advocacy appears in practice guidelines and educational curricula because it is considered to be an essential role of nursing practice even though it may be abstract to teach.

Advocacy is central to the practice of nursing because the actions of the advocate are used to promote the ethical principles upon which modern bioethics is based, including respect for patient autonomy, beneficence, nonmaleficence, and justice (Beauchamp & Childress, 2012). Nursing has a specific role within the context of a therapeutic provider relationship, which places nurses at the interface with patients' needs on a regular basis. While traditional nursing virtues reflect the roles and responsibilities historically embodied within the profession, modern virtues reflect nurses in active advocacy roles. Autonomy, beneficence, nonmaleficence, and justice are central ethical principles inherent within the nursing advocacy role, but Beauchamp and Childress (2012) also described five focal virtues that coincide with these principles in professional clinical practice and are embodied within the clinician's moral character: compassion, discernment, trustworthiness, integrity, and conscientiousness. Advocacy remains the *action* that allows nurses to act on these virtues.

Advocacy Emerging From Other Disciplines

From the public viewpoint, advocacy is often considered from a legal perspective where the definition coincides with the action of pleading the case of another. There is also literature encompassing the term *advocacy* in the sense of either protecting the constitution or protecting people's individual rights (Higginson, 2008). Advocacy groups have emerged across all political and social arenas because of the notion that "the personal is political." As examples, Mothers Against Drunk Driving was founded by a mother whose child was killed by a drunk driver, and hundreds of HIV/AIDS organizations grew out of personal tragedy, loss, and perceived injustices and discrimination of this patient population. Jezewski (1993) added to the definition of advocacy by proposing a model of cultural brokering that has a long history in the discipline of anthropology. *Cultural brokering* is defined as the act of bridging, linking, or mediating between groups of persons of differing cultural backgrounds for the purpose of reducing conflict or producing change. The centrality of culture in this definition coincides with the tenets of the discipline of anthropology.

Interestingly, as London (2008) noted, advocacy in the business literature often overlaps with nursing concepts because advocacy is considered to be a role within corporate social responsibility and entrepreneurship. In business, *advo-*

cacy is defined as the act of supporting an idea, a need, a person, or a group. Furthermore, social advocates in business take public action to engender fair treatment or further the cause of people in need who cannot speak for themselves, where the overall goal is often to promote social welfare. As discussed later in this chapter, some of the philosophical underpinnings of the development of the concept within nursing, specifically oncology nursing, share this definition's attributes. Antecedents for promoting advocacy within the business literature are very goal oriented (i.e., identifying cost and value, sources of support, and adversaries) and still maintain the organization as one of the outcome beneficiaries, which is different from the nurse-oriented focus on the *patient's* well-being as the ultimate beneficiary (London, 2008).

Epistemological Perspective and Ontological Sources

Before understanding the nature and meaning of patient advocacy as conceptualized by the biomedical literature, it is imperative to understand the origin of the term (*ontology*) and theoretical referents (*epistemology*). A review of the literature reveals many definitions for patient advocacy, but the most frequently discussed and earliest nursing models include Curtin's (1979) human advocacy model, Gadow's (1980) theory of existential advocacy, and Kohnke's (1982) functional model of patient advocacy. All of the models include the assertion that advocacy is about helping patients to become clear about what they want (Gadow, 1989). According to Curtin (1979), the end purpose of nursing is the welfare of other human beings, and arguments lead back to the belief in the humanity in each individual, whose entitlement to human rights arises out of human need. Because of a common humanity, "human advocacy" develops, forming the foundation of the nurse–patient relationship. Nurses express the advocacy role by creating an atmosphere that is supportive to patients' decision making, helping them to make sense of the meaning in their living or dying (Curtin, 1979). Curtin also argued that advocacy forms the philosophical foundation of nursing practice, thus perpetuating the notion of advocacy as a role and central tenet to the nursing profession (Curtin, 1979).

Although Gadow (1980) promoted a similar philosophical approach as Curtin, the author differed when she argued that advocacy should not be defined by the role but rather by the philosophical underpinnings. Her theory of existential advocacy is based on the principle that freedom of self-determination is the most fundamental and valuable human right (Gadow, 1980). She asserted that nurses should help patients become clear about what they want by helping them to discern and clarify their values for a particular situation, thereby reaching a decision after expressing their own relevant needs. She warned that taking this approach could negatively lead to paternalism if the nurse is not careful. The biggest barrier to the use of Gadow's and Curtin's philosophical approaches is the difficulty in applying the concepts for use in research and clinical practice.

Kohnke (1982) proposed a functional model of patient advocacy that is more pragmatic in its approach and involves informing patients and then supporting their decisions. She argued that every nurse has a choice to make and must decide whether the nurse wants to advocate and whether the nurse is the best and most-informed person to inform the patient. Kohnke differed from Curtin in her belief that advocacy is not a natural role for nurses to occupy but can be acquired if they accept the role. She also acknowledged that advocacy can be risky and suggested preparatory courses for nurses to help them cope with the potential consequences of taking on this action. A limitation of Kohnke's definition is that it is not significantly different from the concept of informed consent.

The advocacy models of Curtin (1979), Gadow (1980), and Kohnke (1982) all have the same basis in a belief in personal autonomy that means individuals are permitted personal liberty and freedom to determine their own actions. The ontological origin for this combined model of advocacy reflects the application of the theory of humanism. One overriding value in humanism is that of human dignity and the power to reason based on free will (Fagermoen, 2006). Watson's theory of caring often is discussed along with humanism because it provides a foundation for nursing as a moral practice (Fagermoen, 2006). In this context, care is best seen as moral motivation to act in regard to a patient's well-being, respect for the patient as a person, and the patient's inherent worth as an individual regardless of capacity and competence (Fagermoen, 2006). The value of human dignity is core, and autonomy and equality stem from this ethical foundation. Fagermoen (2006) asserted, "Humanism in the new century has to embrace not only the idea that humans must be allowed to exercise the power of self-determination but also at the same time realize that in doing so there is a great danger of alienating ourselves from the basic values of humanity" (p. 180).

The next major addition to the concept of nursing advocacy occurred with works published in the 1980s that expanded the perspective of advocacy to include social advocacy. In 1986, Copp published on the concept of advocacy as it related to vulnerable populations. She wrote, "It is obvious that when individuals lose power to represent themselves, and their needs, wishes, values, and choices, others must advocate for them" (Copp, 1986, p. 255). Although it may not be presented as such, nurses often do represent individuals who may not be in a position to speak from their own point of view. Since then, in practice, empirically based advocacy studies seem to be attached to vulnerable groups such as patients who are emergent or require critical care, terminally ill patients, patients with cancer, children, those lacking the capacity to make decisions, or socially marginalized groups (Vaartio & Leino-Kilpi, 2005). Within this view of advocacy, nurses have a responsibility to empower patients (Copp, 1986). This analysis presumes some level of vulnerability inherent in either the individual patient or the population where nurses can act; thus, vulnerability is a necessary antecedent to nursing advocacy practices. Copp viewed vulnerability as a variable that exists along a continuum and not in a dichotomous fashion. She defined a continuum of vulnerability that included the potentially vulnerable (e.g., an infant who lives in a home with high levels of lead), the circumstantially vulnerable (e.g., those who were previously well but undergo an abrupt situation, such as a trauma), the temporarily vulnerable (e.g., those who are incarcerated), the episodically vulnerable (e.g., individuals with recurrent exacerbations of disease, such as sickle-cell disease), and the permanently vulnerable (e.g., those who have residual damage from disease, such as hemiplegia secondary to stroke) (Copp, 1986). It is important to note this idea of varying degrees of vulnerability because advocacy itself also occurs along a continuum and is not a dichotomous or yes/no event. This illustrates one reason why it has been difficult to build consensus on this concept because the nursing advocacy models depend on individual situations and varying contexts. Advocacy can take a proactive approach when informing patients of choices and providing autonomy as well as a reactive approach if a nurse feels that a patient's basic human rights or ethical tenets have been violated, further complicating its broad definition.

In 1989, Fowler proposed the social advocacy model. This model retained nurses' concerns about individual patients yet advanced them beyond institutional walls and called for participation in social criticism and social change. Social advocacy calls attention to inequalities and inconsistencies in the provision of health care at both the micro- and macrosystem levels and is deeply rooted within the philosophy and ethics of social justice (Fowler, 1989). Social advocacy attempts to correct both clinical and social injustices that fail to respect patients as persons, their rights, their values, or their dignity but broadens the advocacy models of Curtin (1979), Gadow (1980), and Kohnke (1982) to expand nurses' concerns beyond the immediate bedside.

The expansion of the concept of advocacy to include definitions with origins in social justice coincides with the ontological perspective of feminist theory. By using Harding's (1986) inclusion of feminism to comprise socially marginalized groups, vulnerable groups that as a whole have been previously excluded may, in fact, have an epistemological privilege and should be accounted for in practice and research. Feminist theory can be applied to the development of the social justice component of advocacy at either the individual or population level.

Conceptual, Theoretical, and Empirical Applications

Building on the notion that advocacy can be a proactive, reactive, or social justice–based approach, attributes were assigned to each (see Figure 5-1). Proactive forms of nursing advocacy include informing patients so that they can make informed decisions, safeguarding patient rights by providing autonomy and self-determination, empowering patients to make decisions, and serving as patient navigators to help guide patients through complex disease processes or medical stays. Reactive advocacy is centered on the preservation of patient values through mediation between family members and other providers, or if patients become

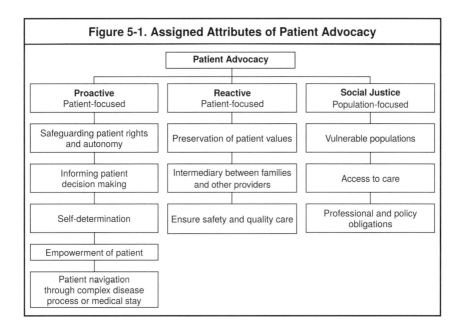

Figure 5-1. Assigned Attributes of Patient Advocacy

unable to speak for themselves. Oftentimes a conflict—or the potential for conflict—is present for this form of advocacy to emerge. The term *whistle-blowing* surfaces in this form of advocacy in the literature, with the goal described as ensuring patient safety and quality care. The attributes of social justice advocacy often are population based instead of patient based and are described as advocating for populations of vulnerable people who are receiving or are at risk for receiving inequities in healthcare delivery. Professional and policy obligations also stem from social justice–based advocacy because a goal is to promote social change and welfare.

Empirical referents are classes or categories of actual phenomena demonstrating the occurrence of the concept of advocacy (Knafl & Deatrick, 2000). Beginning with the theoretical works of Curtin (1979), Gadow (1980), and Kohnke (1982), Table 5-1 illustrates empirical referents for proactive, reactive, and social justice forms of advocacy in general nursing practice. No standardized tool exists that assesses the action of advocacy, but attempts were made to qualitatively ask nurses to describe their experiences of patient advocacy. Additional limitations in the concept were noted for these examples. Proactive forms of patient advocacy in oncology include promoting opportunities in cancer prevention and survivorship, educating patients about genetic testing, understanding preferences for patient involvement in decision making, and tailoring education needs for newly diagnosed patients. Examples of reactive forms of advocacy include supporting refusal of treatment, intervening in cases of inadequate pain management, and supporting end-of-life decisions made by family members. Social justice–based examples of nursing advocacy include nursing involvement in healthcare reform, advocating for equitable access to care, understanding and eliminating disparities in cancer care, and understanding the Oncology Nursing Society's (ONS's) stance as a professional organization and its impact on advocacy.

Table 5-1. Theoretical Attributes and Examples of Patient Advocacy in Nursing

Author	Purpose	Attributes	Empirical Referents	Limitations of Concept
Curtin, 1979	Human advocacy model; considered humanistic	Proactive	Nurses see patients as distinct human beings. Illness affects integrity of person. Human rights and advocacy arise from human needs. Decision making	Lack of ability to operationalize variables Applicability to clinical practice
Gadow, 1980	Existential advocacy; philosophical	Proactive	Self-determination is the most fundamental human right. Nurses should help patients clarify their values. Potential exists for paternalism.	Lack of ability to operationalize variables Applicability to clinical practice
Kohnke, 1982	Functional model of patient advocacy; inclination toward legal advocacy	Proactive	Based on right to self-determination Inform patients, then support the decisions they make.	Simpler model Advocacy can be risky to nurses.
Winslow, 1984	Nurses and patients as partners in advocacy	Reactive	Nurses help patients to overcome barriers to meet their needs. Nurses may have conflicting interests. Critique involving loyalty Often associated with controversy	Offers few suggestions for multiple problems presented Nurses themselves are sometimes powerless.

(Continued on next page)

Table 5-1. Theoretical Attributes and Examples of Patient Advocacy in Nursing (Continued)

Author	Purpose	Attributes	Empirical Referents	Limitations of Concept
Copp, 1986	Ethics of justice	Reactive and social justice	Intervening with vulnerable populations Universal access to adequate nursing and health care	Diverse activities Some nurses may not feel it is their responsibility in this advocacy model because it moves beyond the individual patient and advocates for a population.
Corcoran, 1988	Operationalizing advocacy role	Proactive	Work is based on Curtin (1979) and Gadow (1980). Helping others to decide (created stepwise process)	Is more a slogan rather than truly represented in practice Model has not been tested in clinical practice.
Fowler, 1989	Social advocacy model	Social justice	Rights for individual patients go beyond institution Inequalities Equitable access	Model is potentially too broad; scope is large. Some nurses may not feel that social advocacy is their responsibility because it moves beyond the individual patient and advocates for a population.
Jezewski, 1993	Cultural broker model	Reactive	Bridging and mediating between groups Differences between the cultural system of the patient and healthcare delivery	Anthropologic-based model Only sometimes operationalized in routine clinical nursing practice

(Continued on next page)

Table 5-1. Theoretical Attributes and Examples of Patient Advocacy in Nursing *(Continued)*

Author	Purpose	Attributes	Empirical Referents	Limitations of Concept
Snowball, 1996	Asking nurses about advocating for patients: "proactive and reactive accounts"	Proactive and reactive	Therapeutic relationship must be present; need exists for the nurse to relate to the patient. Specific individual-based advocacy while also seeing need for "bigger picture beyond bedside"	Exploratory study based on a very small sample (15 nurses)
Willard, 1996	Advocacy vs. beneficence	Proactive	Confusion with beneficence Moral status of patient autonomy Obligations owed to patients by nurses How can nurses be supported in this endeavor?	Detracts from level of professionalism because somewhat unattainable
Breier-Mackie, 2001	Can nurses help doctors listen to patients?	Reactive	Explores us vs. them: Do doctors and nurses consider patient autonomy differently? Nurse role as mediator Differences in delivery systems Nurses have awareness and desire for therapeutic communication.	States that delivering autonomy is a moral commitment to all providers, but does not offer tools or suggestions

Developing a Conceptual Model of Patient Advocacy

In an attempt to define and identify the concept of advocacy, a conceptual model for patient advocacy was developed (see Figure 5-2). On the individual-based level of advocacy, a patient's condition and need for advocacy tend to be the most cited reasons for demanding advocacy actions (Bu & Jezewski,

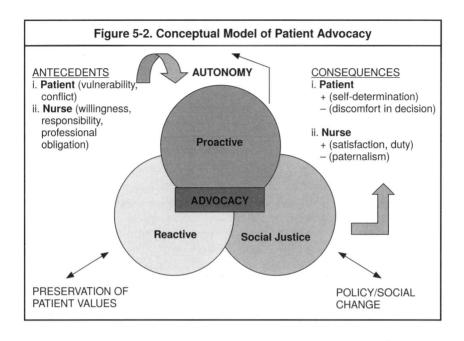

Figure 5-2. Conceptual Model of Patient Advocacy

2006). Patient vulnerability comprises patients who cannot fully represent and protect their own rights, needs, benefits, and wishes, or those who are unable to make or carry out their own decisions (Copp, 1986). Some level of vulnerability should be demonstrated as a necessary antecedent for advocacy. In a reactive advocacy situation, conflict may be present for the nurse to intercede. There are also antecedent variables that the nurse must encompass to fill the role of patient advocate. The nurse must be willing to embody this role, as he or she may see advocacy as a responsibility, a professional obligation, or an altruistic or ethical duty of nursing. The nurse must also have the knowledge, inherent leadership, and communication abilities to carry out the role.

The role of patient advocate has both positive and negative consequences. If the role is carried out successfully, patients may feel empowered or have a renewed sense of self-determination and autonomy. Nurses may also feel personal satisfaction while enhancing the public's perception of nursing and improving professional status (Bu & Jezewski, 2006). In some situations, however, negative repercussions can occur. When given autonomy, patients may feel extreme discomfort in making a decision. Additionally, nurses may encompass a role of advocacy that is overly protective of the patient, and even if nurses think they know what is best for the patient, without giving the patient the ultimate choice, paternalism could result. Advocates also may experience extreme conflict in the form of moral distress and feel powerless to do the right thing or feel institutional constraints in carrying out advocacy roles (Bu & Jezewski, 2006).

Patient advocacy was placed within the context of the nursing role because, although advocacy itself is an action, it is described more uniformly in the literature as a role for which professional nurses should strive. With origins rooted in the ethics of nursing practice, the advocacy role is described as a moral concept that requires a nurse to always actively support the patient (Hamric, 2000). Embedded within the moral construct of advocacy is the axiom that the health of the individual is a social good and valued as a worthy goal (Weed & McKeown, 2003).

Much thought surrounds the notion that social justice should be associated with the role of patient advocacy in oncology nursing, but perhaps it is not a central component, particularly when one believes the nursing role should focus on patient-based proactive and reactive advocacy efforts. To answer this, the public health literature was evaluated for aid in developing the social justice component as it applies to oncology nursing because many of the same charges of using advocacy to promote social responsibility and influence health policy making are shared by clinicians (physicians, nurses), public health professionals (epidemiologists, medical anthropologists), and other members of the healthcare team (social workers, chaplains). Two distinct roles emerged as defined professional responsibilities of those involved in public health: one is defined as professional practice constrained to science and practice, and the other aids active participation in public health policy making (Weed & Mink, 2002). These roles mirror recent trends seen in the nursing literature that promote clinicians' use of knowledge and resources to become social advocates by directly contributing to health policy.

Some argue that those who use science to promote social responsibility and lobby for those with socially defined health problems can bias their interpretation and make them less objective scientists and clinicians. Weed and McKeown (2003) described the defining axiom for public health's approach to problems is the value that the health of the public is a social good they can undertake. Furthermore, clinicians cannot claim to be committed to public health as a social good without accepting the responsibility of ensuring that the knowledge gained in their roles as scientists is used to achieve that good (Weed & McKeown, 2003). Therefore, the idea of using social justice to solve socially based health problems and address vulnerable populations is shared and can be accessed by all health-related disciplines, and should be central to patient advocacy used by oncology nurses.

Case Studies

The following three case studies are based on actual patient encounters and represent each component of the patient advocacy model as directly applied to oncology nursing practice. The first case demonstrates the nurse as a proactive advocate, the second case illustrates reactive advocacy, and the third discusses social justice advocacy. Each case is presented with background literature to provide context and includes a discussion on the role of the nurse as advocate.

Case 1: Proactive Advocacy

Annie Lopez is a 32-year-old woman newly diagnosed with acute myeloid leukemia (AML). Mrs. Lopez and her husband have one child, but she has always envisioned having a large family, and prior to her diagnosis she and her husband were actively trying to conceive their second child. Her oncologist and hematology-oncology nurse practitioner discuss her diagnosis, present treatment options, and a plan to start induction using cytarabine and daunorubicin as soon as possible. Mrs. Lopez and her husband begin to realize the magnitude of the diagnosis. She understands that she needs to begin chemotherapy immediately, but she is most concerned about her current pregnancy status. The nurse practitioner begins scheduling Mrs. Lopez's induction admission and also performs a pregnancy test. When the results come back, Mrs. Lopez and her husband are relieved to learn that she is not currently pregnant, meaning she can go forward with therapy without risk to a fetus. Even though Mrs. Lopez and her husband have already had a long day in the clinic, the nurse performs education on future fertility considerations, which Mrs. Lopez did not realize was a potential issue. Mrs. Lopez's chemotherapy regimens fall under a lower risk profile for impact on future fertility, but even so, it could potentially be an issue for them later. Mrs. Lopez and her husband are thankful for the information, and she feels more certain about her decision to move forward with chemotherapy induction.

With a renewed focus on cancer survivorship and late effects of treatment within the past decade, more attention has been placed on the risk of cancer-related infertility as a result of treatment. The American Society of Clinical Oncology has published guidelines to address infertility risks associated with various treatment modalities (Lee et al., 2006). Many cancer treatment agents used in the adolescent and young adult age groups are associated with premature ovarian failure in women and decreased sperm production in men (Lee et al., 2006). In a study to determine the risk of treatment-related menopause after treatment of premenopausal women with chemotherapy, the risk of menopause one year after diagnosis was found to be 50% among women aged 40 and younger (Goodwin, Ennis, Pritchard, Trudeau, & Hood, 1999).

Is infertility a necessary price to pay for cancer survival? To date, most insurance companies do not offer assisted reproductive techniques as covered benefits. For young women, fertility preservation has proved to be a more difficult feat with larger economic and feasibility barriers. Embryo cryopreservation is considered to be an established method of fertility preservation but requires a partner or sperm donor, a delay in cancer treatment by about four to six weeks because of the time required for ovarian stimulation (with daily injections of follicle-stimulating hormone), and out-of-pocket costs ranging from $10,000 to $12,000 (Lee et al., 2006). Because of the emergent nature of fertility preservation techniques and the possibility of a resulting embryo if cryopreservation is used, the decision to pursue this option is also fraught with ethical implications. What happens to the embryo if the woman does not survive? What if the woman has a very dismal prognosis? Is it ethical to delay treatment in order for a woman to take the time to pursue fertility preservation? These ethical issues may inhibit providers from encouraging fertility preservation assistance (Robertson, 2005).

From a practice perspective, the available evidence suggests that fertility preservation and counseling are of great importance to young adults diagnosed with cancer (Lee et al., 2006). Even so, recent surveys of cancer survivors of reproductive age concur that at least half of the participants had no memory of a discussion of fertility at the time of their treatment (Duffy, Allen, & Clark, 2005; Schover, Brey, Lichtin, Lipshultz, & Jeha, 2002; Zebrack, Casillas, Nohr, Adams, & Zeltzer, 2004). Even when patients do recall infertility discussions, many are not satisfied with the quality and amount of information provided. Partridge et al. (2004) concluded that young women with early-stage breast cancer were more likely to choose a less-toxic chemotherapy regimen given the choice and knowledge that it would not inhibit fertility, regardless of the fact that it conferred slightly less protection from recurrence, indicating that fertility-related knowledge does affect treatment decisions made by women and their partners.

In Mrs. Lopez's case, the nurse's role as a proactive advocate may seem like an intuitive one. Although patient education and guidance with decision making are natural and everyday nursing occurrences, such a case of proactive advocacy demonstrates the nurse educating on a complicated topic that is extremely important to the patient. The day of diagnosis is an emotionally challenging one for patients, and the amount of education provided about the diagnosis and treatment regimens can be overwhelming. Additionally, with a diagnosis of AML, not much time is available to process decisions before beginning induction. Nurses have described that starting a conversation about fertility can be difficult because of the gravity of the diagnosis and the notion that fertility preservation (particularly in women) is a very costly and time-sensitive endeavor that may not be available to all patients. Because it is not a central aspect of a curative approach to treatment, fertility counseling can be easy to overlook. Researchers have demonstrated that despite these circumstances, patients still want to be informed of potential fertility risks and options to preserve fertility, if necessary. By listening to Mrs. Lopez's narrative and current priorities, her nurse was able to deliver information that would ultimately empower Mrs. Lopez in moving forward with her treatment plan.

Case 2: Reactive Advocacy

Thomas Gee is a 76-year-old man with large B-cell lymphoma. His disease persisted despite multiple chemotherapy regimens, and his malignancy recently progressed while he was receiving radiation therapy. Each week in clinic, his physical condition rapidly declines as a result of his disease, cachexia, and impaired nutritional intake. Mr. Gee remains subdued and flat in his expression. The student nurse notes Mr. Gee's rapid physical and emotional deterioration and asks the physician whether he wants to initiate a palliative care consult, given that the patient is exhibiting many distressing symptoms and his physical and psychological states have been declining. The physician states, "The family isn't ready to hear about that yet," and wants to try one more chemotherapy modality to see if it has any palliative effects. Upon hearing that Mr. Gee will be scheduled for a different chemotherapy regimen, the family gets excited about trying a new approach, with some family members stating that this will "build him back up." The family is not aware of the magnitude of Mr. Gee's current disease state and believes there is a chance for a complete response with this new chemotherapy.

Because of intense and prolonged treatment regimens, patients with hematologic malignancies nonresponsive to treatment often experience high levels of cancer-related distress (Albrecht & Rosenzweig, 2012). Distress has been found to occur in almost 50% of patients with advanced hematologic malignancies, and signs may manifest as anger, sadness, insomnia, anorexia, and social isolation (Carlson et al., 2004). At this stage in the cancer trajectory, patients often have unmet needs in various domains that propagate their distress, including issues with the structure and process of care (coordination across healthcare disciplines and settings); physical symptoms; psychological (depression, anxiety), social (familial and other relationships of support network), spiritual, and existential aspects of care; cultural considerations; end-of-life care considerations; and ethical and legal aspects of care (advance care planning) (Dahlin, 2013). Within the past decade, the concept of palliative care has shifted to incorporate these domains early in the disease trajectory, and the relevance for this type of expertise in the context of metastatic or unresponsive cancer has been recognized (Gaertner, Wolf, & Voltz, 2012).

Clinicians who care for patients with advanced cancer are tasked with providing symptom control, initiating conversations about realistic therapeutic goals, coordinating care delivery, and addressing appropriate end-of-life care concerns while simultaneously managing the curative approach until patients are transitioned to comfort and hospice care (Gaertner et al., 2012). Those who specialize in palliative care can alleviate some of this burden because of the discipline's focus on symptom management, psychosocial care, support in decision making, and the potential to improve quality of care delivery while also providing cost-effective medical care (Temel et al., 2010). Palliative care has traditionally been linked to hospice or end-of-life care and thus is delivered late in the course of disease, often only to patients who are hospitalized on inpatient units (Temel et al., 2010). To have a meaningful impact on a patient's disease trajectory, palliative care services must be provided early in the course of the disease and incorporate those patients managed on an outpatient basis (Temel et al., 2010).

Providing quality care for patients with advanced cancer requires a vast amount of professional resources (Gaertner et al., 2012). In the case of Mr. Gee, the student nurse initiated the appropriate first step in making a patient-based assessment of distress based on physical, psychological, and knowledge deficits. She then acted as a reactive advocate when she voiced her concerns to the attending physician caring for Mr. Gee. In this situation, the reactive advocate was focused on delivering coordinated quality care to Mr. Gee and most notably prompting a discussion between the clinicians and family regarding therapeutic goals of care. Although the family agreed to move forward with a new chemotherapy, it is very clear that they were not aware of the clinical intent of this palliative endeavor. Additionally, Mr. Gee's current psychological state made it difficult to understand his goals of care, and an advocate would work to understand and preserve his values. The ultimate goal for Mr. Gee would be a consult to palliative care services, which ideally would have occurred as soon as distress began. Although student nurses may likely feel limited in their emerging role as advocate, they are often able to witness clinical situations unfold with limited biases and a fresh perspective. In this particular case, the student nurse was able to speak at length with the attending physician and nurse practitioner about her perspective of the case, which prompted a palliative care consult and provided significant education regarding therapeutic goals of care and prognosis.

Case 3: Social Justice Advocacy

Chris Jackson is a 19-year-old young adult being treated for relapsed osteosarcoma on the pediatric hematology-oncology floor. He is very enthusiastic about completing his physical therapy today because he wants to "look good" for his girlfriend who is planning a visit later that afternoon. Mr. Jackson tells his nurse that it has been very difficult to see his girlfriend lately because he had to move into his grandparents' house several hours away from her and the hospital. Knowing that his mom is very involved in his care, the nurse inquires about the move. Mr. Jackson explains that after he withdrew from college and lost his student health insurance, he was unable to obtain health insurance independently because of his cancer. (His mother works part time but is uninsured herself.) Because his mother exceeds the poverty-level cutoff needed to qualify for Medicaid, Mr. Jackson had to move in with his grandparents so he was able to qualify for Medicaid independently. The move has drastically affected his quality of life because he is hours away from his friends, girlfriend, and mother, as well as the hospital where he is being treated. He is unsure when he will be able to move back in with his mother.

Young adults aged 19–29 represent the largest under- and uninsured group in the United States (Collins & Nicolson, 2009). Schoen, Collins, Kriss, and Doty (2008) reported that 59% of all young adults in this age bracket were either underinsured or not insured for the entire year (i.e., they had gaps in insurance coverage). Because insurance coverage for this demographic is often based on employment or student status, and adolescent and young adult patients with cancer face enhanced difficulty with maintaining employment or entrance to higher education, the confluence of these factors makes it even more difficult to maintain health insurance after diagnosis. This coincides with the "aging out" of childhood health plans for young adults who may have recently been covered under their parents' insurance plans (Bleyer & Barr, 2007).

Uninsured patients with cancer have historically had a difficult time obtaining health insurance after their diagnosis because of the cancer being classified as a preexisting condition (Virgo, Burkhardt, Cokkinides, & Ward, 2010). The American Cancer Society recently polled individuals with cancer younger than age 65 and found that 34% were uninsured or underinsured for a period of time following their diagnosis, and approximately 59% of those who were uninsured could not afford to purchase insurance (Virgo et al., 2010). In another study, up to 25% of cancer survivors had difficulty obtaining insurance or had exclusion clauses pertaining to a cancer diagnosis, compared to 1%–3% of age-matched controls (Langeveld et al., 2003). Similarly, in a follow-up report of childhood survivors by the Childhood Cancer Survivor Study, 30% had difficulty in obtaining insurance coverage (Nagarajan et al., 2003). Finally, in a study of adult survivors of acute lymphoblastic leukemia, 28.4% had been denied health insurance and 18.6% reported facing unmanageable premiums (Pui et al., 2003). The hypothesis remains that lack of insurance decreases therapeutic options available to patients, such as access to second opinions, access to expensive treatment and medication, lack of participation in clinical trials, and limited choice of specialists. State-run and state- and federally funded Medicaid is an option for some who are younger than age 65; however, only select segments of the poor (particularly those older than age 18) qualify for Medicaid and must meet criteria based on having income less than 133% of the federal poverty level (Virgo et al., 2010).

Passed as law in 2010 and upheld by the U.S. Supreme Court in 2012, the ACA has been the most sweeping healthcare reform since the formation of Medicare and Medicaid in 1965. One of the first implemented provisions of the ACA permits young adults up to the age of 26 to obtain health insurance as dependents on a parent's private health plan (Cantor, Monheit, DeLia, & Lloyd, 2012). Additionally, the preexisting condition limits that inhibited many patients with cancer from even qualifying for private healthcare insurance are now addressed under the ACA, and patients with preexisting conditions who were uninsured for at least six months are now eligible for subsidized coverage (no less than 65% of medical costs) through national high-risk insurance pools (Bleyer, 2010). Even this condition still presents challenges because it assumes a period of uninsurance to qualify for the national high-risk pool; a six-month period of cancer treatment is enough to bankrupt many patients. Finally, many but not all states are in the process of expanding Medicaid eligibility criteria so that more low-income individuals can enroll. In 2014, patients without access to insurance through Medicaid, Medicare, or their employer began purchasing coverage through state- or region-based health exchanges (Virgo et al., 2010).

In Mr. Jackson's case, the role of the nurse advocate likely went beyond advocating for an individual and moved to advocating for a cause or population (in this case, the under- or uninsured or advocacy for more comprehensive healthcare reform). Mr. Jackson was finally able to obtain access to Medicaid but in doing so gave up some of his independence and quality of life. Navigating through coverage hurdles was not an easy process for him or his family and likely had negative psychosocial and access-to-treatment–related impacts. In Mr. Jackson's case, nurses could use social advocacy to tell his story and advocate for change related to health policy and insurance coverage.

Implications for Nursing Practice

Isn't Patient Advocacy Just Good Nursing Care?

It can be argued that applying patient advocacy in both clinical practice and research is nursing's moral obligation and professional responsibility. Contemporary ethical theories classify behaviors and actions as either "obligation" or "beyond obligation," with actions beyond obligation being the pursuit of an exceptional but optional ideal (Beauchamp & Childress, 2012). A continuum exists between strict obligation (the core demands in common morality) through weaker obligations (the periphery of ordinary expectations) to ideals beyond obligatory, ending with higher-level actions beyond obligation (acts of supreme self-sacrifice). Thinking about patient advocacy across this continuum is a helpful practice for the application of patient advocacy within the scope of nurses' daily professional environments. Consider different examples of advocacy that are routinely encountered, such as finding someone to walk with a patient to the outpatient pharmacy at discharge, or working to coordinate a procedure on a day that coincides with a patient already being in the clinic. These actions may seem like just "good nursing care," but in reality they go beyond strict moral obligations of nursing care. Other examples of proactive and reactive advocacy may also fall into the classification of good nursing care, but in truth they are not actions of strict professional obligation and do exceed basic requirements to coincide with ideals beyond obligation.

Social justice components of advocacy have been described as the foundational moral perspective of public health and the basis for subsequent care of vulnerable populations (Powers & Faden, 2006). Historically, nursing has championed many issues of social justice, such as homelessness, poverty, addiction, housing quality, rural healthcare delivery, and violence assessment (Paquin, 2011). Social justice aspects of advocacy often are viewed slightly differently than proactive and reactive patient-based advocacy efforts because they are more difficult to conceptualize within the scope of routine nursing practice. Nurses are confronted with the realities of social inequities on a regular basis, yet they may feel frustrated that they do not have time within the day to act on behalf of a group or specific population. Giving voice to specific concerns of certain groups is a natural fit for advocacy in the health policy arena. There are ethical assumptions and implications for all health policies and ethical applications to the process itself (Churchill, 2002).

How Can Nurses Become Patient Advocates?

Listen and share patient stories (in a way that protects their identity). Humanizing patients' stories and experiences is a natural way that nurses can become involved in advocacy efforts. Nurses have many incredible stories to tell. By speaking on behalf of patients or writing their stories in a meaningful way, nurses can add to the shared understanding of their experiences and struggles. For example, the popular column "Narrative Matters" in the journal *Health Affairs* gives clinicians the opportunity to share stories that have relevant and timely policy implications. Politicians often use such stories to advocate for certain health policies because they provide an easier way of connecting to a cause. Statistics and numbers can highlight certain aspects, but a narrative-based approach to sharing patient stories allows the cause to have a "face" and thus more meaning. In addition to journals that publish these types of columns, nurses can share advocacy narratives via newspapers, magazines, and online blogs.

Use evidence-based practice and join practice committees. Some might not connect evidence-based practice to advocacy, but getting involved in practice committees and striving to provide the highest quality nursing care is a natural fit for advocacy efforts. Always approaching evidence-based nursing care as the gold standard allows nurses to provide quality care while staying informed on issues specific to the populations of interest. By continuing to acquire this knowledge, nurses can effectively translate that care to patients.

Network with others who are interested in advocacy initiatives through social media or nursing organizations. Connecting with other nurses has become increasingly easier via social media sites such as Twitter and Facebook and nursing-focused websites. Professional nursing organizations often are a natural place to connect and get involved in various advocacy efforts. For example, ONS offers a Health Policy Agenda and many other advocacy tools and resources through its website at www.ons.org/advocacy-policy. Nurses are encouraged to view the agenda and other resources and find a way to join a cause that is meaningful to them.

Become involved with nursing legislative days. Many nursing societies and state nursing associations participate in legislative days where members can take their issues of interest directly to people in positions that influence and make policy. Nurses can take advantage of opportunities to travel to state capitals or Washington, DC, and actively engage in the policy-making process, advocating on behalf of specific populations or aspects of nursing practice. As policy work is becoming more central to issues of social justice and advocacy, an increasingly urgent need exists for nurses to engage in policy change (Montgomery, 2012; Spenceley, Reutter, & Allen, 2006).

Incorporate advocacy into nursing education. For patient advocacy to continue to be a component of ethical nursing practice, a sustained focus is necessary. Content about advocacy and nursing needs to be tailored and introduced into curricula for nursing students at every level. Skills such as understanding how to advocate for individual patients and populations of interest, communicating about health policy, and applying advocacy to the nursing role need to be introduced and taught as early as possible in schools of nursing, both theoretically and in clinical practice.

Conclusion

There has never been a more pressing time in history for oncology nurses to become patient advocates and apply this concept into their everyday practice and professional responsibility. Nurses work on the front lines of patient care delivery, regularly overcoming barriers to respond effectively to the rapidly changing healthcare system (Institute of Medicine [IOM], 2011). They also have become organized in delivering unified responses to inequity to maximize care delivery for vulnerable populations. Nurses have played a vital role in advocating for healthcare reform and are now tasked with implementing the 2010 passage of the ACA—the broadest reform of healthcare coverage and delivery since the creation of Medicare and Medicaid in 1965 (IOM, 2011).

The IOM report *The Future of Nursing* outlined four key areas of focus for the future of the profession: (a) nurses practicing to the fullest extent of their education and training, (b) nurses achieving higher levels of training through seamless academic progression, (c) nurses being full partners with physicians and other members of the healthcare team in redesigning health care in the United States, and (d) better data collection and improved information infrastructures for effective workforce planning and policy making (IOM, 2011). By striving to meet each of these outlined goals, nurses will be able to better incorporate activities that allow for patient advocacy within the context of their professional practice and educational development.

Given this framework and understanding, it is imperative to further operationalize the concept of patient advocacy for knowledge development and dissemination. Until advocacy can be defined systematically and objectively, measuring a nurse's impact in a given situation, both in practice and in research endeavors, is difficult. Patient advocacy is a lens for understanding moral actions inherent in nursing care. The qualitative empirical work that has already been done needs to be expanded to include larger sample sizes and more diverse advocacy activities. Knowledge development in these areas will shed light on how nurses can best develop specific interventions that can be used within ethical and decision-making frameworks, as well as in the context of vulnerable populations.

References

Albrecht, T.A., & Rosenzweig, M. (2012). Management of cancer-related distress in patients with a hematologic malignancy. *Journal of Hospice and Palliative Nursing, 14,* 462–468. doi:10.1097/NJH.0b013e318268d04e

Annas, G.J., & Healey, J. (1974). The patient rights advocate. *Journal of Nursing Administration, 4*(3), 25–31.

Baldwin, M.A. (2003). Patient advocacy: A concept analysis. *Nursing Standard, 17*(21), 33–39.

Beauchamp, T.L., & Childress, J.F. (2012). *Principles of biomedical ethics* (7th ed.). New York, NY: Oxford University Press.

Bleyer, W.A. (2010). Potential favorable impact of the Affordable Care Act of 2010 on cancer in young adults in the United States. *Cancer Journal, 16,* 563–571. doi:10.1097/PPO.0b013e3181ff6509

Bleyer, W.A., & Barr, R.D. (Eds.). (2007). *Cancer in adolescents and young adults*. New York, NY: Springer.

Breier-Mackie, S. (2001). Patient autonomy and medical paternity: Can nurses help doctors to listen to patients? *Nursing Ethics, 8*, 510–521. doi:10.1177/096973300100800605

Bu, X., & Jezewski, M.A. (2006). Developing a mid-range theory of patient advocacy through concept analysis. *Journal of Advanced Nursing, 57*, 101–110. doi:10.1111/j.1365-2648.2006.04096.x

Cantor, J.C., Monheit, A.C., DeLia, D., & Lloyd, K. (2012). Early impact of the Affordable Care Act on health insurance coverage of young adults. *Health Services Research, 47*, 1773–1790. doi:10.1111/j.1475-6773.2012.01458.x

Carlson, L.E., Angen, M., Cullum, J., Goodey, E., Koopmans, J., Lamont, L., ... Bultz, B.D. (2004). High levels of untreated distress and fatigue in cancer patients. *British Journal of Cancer, 90*, 2297–2304. doi:10.1038/sj.bjc.6601887

Churchill, L.R. (2002). What ethics can contribute to health policy. In M. Danis, C. Clancy, & L.R. Churchill (Eds.), *Ethical dimensions of health policy* (pp. 51–64). New York, NY: Oxford University Press.

Collins, S.R., & Nicolson, J.L. (2009). Young, uninsured and seeking change: Health coverage of young adults and their views on health reform. Findings from the Commonwealth Fund Survey of Young Adults. Retrieved from http://www.commonwealthfund.org/~/media/files/publications/issue-brief/2009/dec/1355_nicholson_young_adults_ib_1218.pdf

Copp, L.A. (1986). The nurse as advocate for vulnerable persons. *Journal of Advanced Nursing, 11*, 255–263. doi:10.1111/j.1365-2648.1986.tb01246.x

Corcoran, S. (1988). Toward operationalizing an advocacy role. *Journal of Professional Nursing, 4*, 242–248. doi:10.1016/S8755-7223(88)80009-7

Curtin, L.L. (1979). The nurse as advocate: Philosophical foundations for nursing. *Advances in Nursing Science, 1*(3), 1–10.

Dahlin, C. (Ed.). (2013). *Clinical practice guidelines for quality palliative care* (3rd ed.). Retrieved from http://www.nationalconsensusproject.org/NCP_Clinical_Practice_Guidelines_3rd_Edition.pdf

Duffy, C.M., Allen, S.M., & Clark, M.A. (2005). Discussions regarding reproductive health for young women with breast cancer undergoing chemotherapy. *Journal of Clinical Oncology, 23*, 766–773. doi:10.1200/JCO.2005.01.134

Fagermoen, M.S. (2006). Humanism in nursing theory: A focus on caring. In H.S. Kim & I. Kollak (Eds.), *Nursing theories: Conceptual and philosophical foundations* (2nd ed., pp. 157–183). New York, NY: Springer.

Fowler, M.D. (1989). Social advocacy: Ethical issues in critical care. *Heart and Lung, 18*, 97–99.

Gadow, S. (1980). Existential advocacy: Philosophical foundation of nursing. In S.F. Spicker & S. Gadow (Eds.), *Nursing, images and ideals: Opening dialogue with the humanities* (pp. 79–101). New York, NY: Springer.

Gadow, S. (1989). An ethical case for patient self-determination. *Seminars in Oncology Nursing, 5*, 99–101. doi:10.1016/0749-2081(89)90067-3

Gaertner, J., Wolf, J., & Voltz, R. (2012). Early palliative care for patients with metastatic cancer. *Current Opinion in Oncology, 24*, 357–362. doi:10.1097/CCO.0b013e328352ea20

Goodwin, P.J., Ennis, M., Pritchard, K.I., Trudeau, M., & Hood, N. (1999). Risk of menopause during the first year after breast cancer diagnosis. *Journal of Clinical Oncology, 17*, 2365–2370.

Hamric, A.B. (2000). What is happening to advocacy? *Nursing Outlook, 48*, 103–104. doi:10.1067/mno.2000.107644

Harding, S.G. (1986). *The science question in feminism*. Ithaca, NY: Cornell University Press.

Higginson, S.A. (2008). Constitutional advocacy explains constitutional outcomes. *Florida Law Review, 60*, 857–894.

Institute of Medicine. (2011). *The future of nursing: Leading change, advancing health*. Washington, DC: National Academies Press.

International Council of Nurses. (2012). *ICN code of ethics for nurses*. Geneva, Switzerland: Author.

Jezewski, M.A. (1993). Culture brokering as a model for advocacy. *Nursing and Health Care, 12*, 78–85.

Knafl, K.A., & Deatrick, J.A. (2000). Knowledge synthesis and concept development in nursing. In B.L. Rodgers & K.A. Knafl (Eds.), *Concept development in nursing: Foundations, techniques, and applications* (pp. 39–54). Philadelphia, PA: Saunders.

Kohnke, M.F. (1982). Advocacy: What is it? *Nursing and Health Care, 3,* 314–318.

Langeveld, N.E., Ubbink, M.C., Last, B.F., Grootenhuis, M.A., Voûte, P.A., & de Haan, R.J. (2003). Educational achievement, employment and living situation in long-term young adult survivors of childhood cancer in the Netherlands. *Psycho-Oncology, 12,* 213–225. doi:10.1002/pon.628

Lee, S.J., Schover, L.R., Partridge, A.H., Patrizio, P., Wallace, W.H., Hagerty, K., ... Oktay, K. (2006). American Society of Clinical Oncology recommendations on fertility preservation in cancer patients. *Journal of Clinical Oncology, 24,* 2917–2931. doi:10.1200/JCO.2006.06.5888

London, M. (2008). Leadership and advocacy: Dual roles for corporate social responsibility and social entrepreneurship. *Organizational Dynamics, 37,* 313–326. doi:10.1016/j.orgdyn.2008.07.003

Mallik, M. (1997). Advocacy in nursing—A review of the literature. *Journal of Advanced Nursing, 25,* 130–138. doi:10.1046/j.1365-2648.1997.1997025130.x

Montgomery, T.M. (2012). Visiting Capitol Hill: Tips for meeting with your elected officials. *Nursing for Women's Health, 16,* 369–371. doi:10.1111/j.1751-486X.2012.01760.x

Nagarajan, R., Neglia, J.P., Clohisy, D.R., Yasui, Y., Greenberg, M., Hudson, M., ... Robison, L.L. (2003). Education, employment, insurance, and marital status among 694 survivors of pediatric lower extremity bone tumors: A report from the Childhood Cancer Survivor Study. *Cancer, 97,* 2554–2564. doi:10.1002/cncr.11363

Paquin, S.O. (2011). Social justice advocacy in nursing: What is it? How do we get there? *Creative Nursing, 17,* 63–67. doi:10.1891/1078-4535.17.2.63

Partridge, A.H., Gelber, S., Peppercorn, J., Sampson, E., Knudsen, K., Laufer, M., ... Winer, E.P. (2004). Web-based survey of fertility issues in young women with breast cancer. *Journal of Clinical Oncology, 22,* 4174–4183. doi:10.1200/JCO.2004.01.159

Powers, M., & Faden, R.R. (2006). Social justice and public health. In J. Harris & S. Holm (Eds.), *Social justice: The moral foundations of public health and health policy* (pp. 80–99). New York, NY: Oxford University Press.

Pui, C.-H., Cheng, C., Leung, W., Rai, S.N., Rivera, G.K., Sandlund, J.T., ... Hudson, M.M. (2003). Extended follow-up of long-term survivors of childhood acute lymphoblastic leukemia. *New England Journal of Medicine, 349,* 640–649. doi:10.1056/NEJMoa035091

Robertson, J.A. (2005). Cancer and fertility: Ethical and legal challenges. *Journal of the National Cancer Institute Monographs, 2005*(34), 104–106. doi:10.1093/jncimonographs/lgi008

Schoen, C., Collins, S.R., Kriss, J.L., & Doty, M.M. (2008). How many are underinsured? Trends among U.S. adults, 2003 and 2007. *Health Affairs, 27,* w298–w309. doi:10.1377/hlthaff.27.4.w298

Schover, L.R., Brey, K., Lichtin, A., Lipshultz, L.I., & Jeha, S. (2002). Knowledge and experience regarding cancer, infertility, and sperm banking in younger male survivors. *Journal of Clinical Oncology, 20,* 1880–1889. doi:10.1200/JCO.2002.07.175

Snowball, J. (1996). Asking nurses about advocating for patients: 'Reactive' and 'proactive' accounts. *Journal of Advanced Nursing, 24,* 67–75.

Spenceley, S.M., Reutter, L., & Allen, M.N. (2006). The road less traveled: Nursing advocacy at the policy level. *Policy, Politics and Nursing Practice, 7,* 180–194. doi:10.1177/1527154406293683

Sutor, J.A. (1993). Ethics: Can nurses be effective advocates? *Nursing Standard, 7*(22), 30–32.

Temel, J.S., Greer, J.A., Muzikansky, M.A., Gallagher, E.R., Admane, S., Jackson, V.A., ... Lynch, T.J. (2010). Early palliative care for patients with metastatic non–small-cell lung cancer. *New England Journal of Medicine, 363,* 733–742. doi:10.1056/NEJMoa1000678

Vaartio, H., & Leino-Kilpi, H. (2005). Nursing advocacy—A review of the empirical research 1990–2003. *International Journal of Nursing Studies, 42,* 705–714. doi:10.1016/j.ijnurstu.2004.10.005

Virgo, K.S., Burkhardt, E.A., Cokkinides, V.E., & Ward, E.M. (2010). Impact of health care reform legislation on uninsured and Medicaid-insured cancer patients. *Cancer Journal, 16,* 577–583. doi:10.1097/PPO.0b013e31820189cb

Weed, D.L., & McKeown, R.E. (2003). Science and social responsibility of public health. *Environmental Health Perspectives, 111,* 1804–1808.

Weed, D.L., & Mink, P.J. (2002). Roles and responsibilities of epidemiologists. *Annals of Epidemiology, 12,* 67–72. doi:10.1016/S1047-2797(01)00302-7

Willard, C. (1996). The nurse's role as patient advocate: Obligation or imposition? *Journal of Advanced Nursing, 24,* 60–66. doi:10.1046/j.1365-2648.1996.01698.x

Winslow, G.R. (1984). From loyalty to advocacy: A new metaphor for nursing. *Hastings Center Report, 14*(3), 32–40.

Zebrack, B.J., Casillas, J., Nohr, L., Adams, H., & Zeltzer, L.K. (2004). Fertility issues for young adult survivors of childhood cancer. *Psycho-Oncology, 13,* 689–699. doi:10.1002/pon.784

CHAPTER 6

Communication and Ethics

Lisa Kennedy Sheldon, PhD, APRN-BC, AOCNP®, ANP-BC, and
Dany M. Hilaire, PhD, RN

Introduction

Communication is the foundation of patient-centered oncology care (Epstein & Street, 2007). In cancer care, nurses spend extended periods of time with patients and families in outpatient, inpatient, and homecare settings. This time provides opportunities to communicate with patients and families about many issues, including their beliefs, concerns, and priorities. With clinical experience, oncology nurses develop expert communication skills that are effective, compassionate, and flexible. Discussions with patients and families deepen nurses' understanding about patients' values, cultural backgrounds, and relationships that provide vital information when exploring situations with ethical implications. In addition, nurses serve as patient advocates on an interprofessional team of healthcare providers and advocate for patients during complex decisions. The nurse's role is central to maintaining open lines of communication among the patient, family, and members of the oncology team during complex situations.

The effective use of communication skills is necessary to establish a relationship with patients and families and develop trust, a key component of ethical communication. The establishment of the nurse–patient relationship is a conscious commitment on the part of both parties. The patient has to trust his or her healthcare providers even before care begins. This concept, *unavoidable trust*, creates tension and vulnerability in patients requiring services in healthcare settings (Butts, 2013). It also creates a power differential where nurses and other healthcare providers have more power in the relationship. Nurses respond to this trust by committing to do their best for and with their patients. The patient's trust and the nurse's commitment combine to form the foundation for communication.

To be effective communicators, nurses need an understanding of the basic concepts of communication. Communication is a two-way process of sending and receiving information (McIntyre & Salas, 1995). Problems in communication may occur on many levels, especially in complex situations. Many problems are rooted in the assumption that communication actually has occurred. Effective communication entails accurate sending and receiving of information but also requires a final step: assessment of the received information. This final step ensures that the message was received and interpreted as intended by the sender. For example, in nursing, the "teach-back" method often is used to allow patients to demonstrate the acquisition of skills such as self-injection of medication. During more complex scenarios, senders or speakers may ask receivers their understanding of what was said to ensure that the received message accurately reflects the speaker's intent. This feedback loop has been used in the airline industry to increase accuracy of communication and has subsequently increased safety.

Nurses play a central role in improving communication, promoting safe and ethical care, and advocating for patients and families. Key guidelines for this communication emanate from ethical principles as well as institutional, professional, and legal standards to guide communication and practice. This chapter will review the foundations of nursing communication with the application of ethical principles for nurses working in cancer care.

Basic Concepts of Communication

Nurses learn to communicate with patients and families during undergraduate education and then develop their communication style during independent clinical practice. The primary goal of the nurse–patient relationship is the health, well-being, and safety of the patient (American Nurses Association [ANA], 2015). Together, nurses and patients decide on appropriate interventions based on the best evidence-based practice and an understanding of professional standards, ethical principles, patient rights, institutional standards, and legal statutes. Further clarification of terms and roles is necessary because of the vulnerability of patients and the unequal power differential.

Nurse–Patient Relationship

Nurses, other healthcare providers, and the literature often use the words *healthcare consumer*, *client*, and *patient* to describe one who seeks or receives health care. *Healthcare consumer* is used to describe a person who purchases healthcare services from a healthcare provider. The more commonly used terms *client* and *patient* have slightly different meanings and benefit from further definition. *Merriam-Webster's Collegiate Dictionary* provided the following definitions.

- Client: One who is under the protection of another, or a person who engages the professional advice or services of another. ("Client," n.d.)
- Patient: An individual awaiting or under medical care or treatment, or one that is acted upon; derived from "one who suffers." ("Patient," n.d.)

People who need health care are often in vulnerable positions that require levels of trust and vigilance from healthcare providers. For example, a person may be medicated, in pain, unconscious, or anesthetized and have limited ability to make decisions while in a compromised state. In these situations, nurses and other healthcare providers often are asked to make decisions in a patient's best interests. In this case, the person is under the protection of another, or a *client*. On the other hand, a person may be acted upon for the provision of direct care, the definition of a *patient*.

People trust healthcare providers to act on their behalf through actions such as providing care, delivering treatment to promote health, and sharing the necessary information to permit independent decision making. Patients have a level of vulnerability that is very different from other services provided for clients, such as legal advice or a haircut. For example, most clients in non-healthcare settings are conscious and free from suffering when they receive services from a lawyer or barber. However, with patients, there is a level of vulnerability and the higher stakes of health care, especially cancer care, with life-altering implications.

In cancer care, nurses are called upon to help patients and families adjust and adapt to the diagnosis and treatment of cancer. They assess and support patients during challenging conversations and interpret information to assist in coping, decision making, adjustment, or achieving a peaceful death. Given the vulnerability of patients, nurses assume important responsibilities with moral obligations. While acknowledging that patients are also protected, the term *patient* better symbolizes the vulnerability of care recipients and the responsibility of nurses in providing the best possible care.

Nursing, as an interaction phenomenon, is not only a process of observation and intervention but also the active engagement of nurses with their patients. Nursing theorist Hildegard Peplau (1952, 1992) was the first to develop an interpersonal model of nursing practice, moving away from what nurses do *to* patients and toward what nurses do *with* patients. Working with patients requires excellent communication skills to give and receive information, teach necessary health behaviors, and provide supportive care. Ethically, Peplau's conceptualization of nursing engagement with patients demonstrates more respect for patients (respect for persons) and increases the value of the nurse–patient relationship in developing trust and providing information (truth telling), and supporting patient decision making (autonomy). Many ethical principles, including respect for persons, truth telling, and self-determination and autonomy, are also fundamental components of the nurse–patient relationship.

Respect for Persons

Respect for persons has long been held as an ethical principle with particular relevance for communication in nursing and health care. According to the Belmont Report, respect for persons has two moral requirements: acknowledgment of the autonomy of individuals and acknowledgment of the need to protect those with diminished autonomy (National Commission for the Protection of Human Subjects of Biomedical and Behavioral Research, 1979). However, in another definition, psychoanalyst Carl Rogers defined *respect* or *unconditional positive regard* as the ability to accept despite one's own personal feelings (Rogers, 1961). Acceptance does not mean approval or agreement. It is a nonjudgmental attitude about the patient as a whole person.

Nurses demonstrate respect in many ways when caring for patients with cancer. Patients respond to health or the challenges of illness and treatment based on personal ways of adapting to challenges. Each patient requires respect and acceptance as a unique human being with abilities to cope with these changes in health and functioning. The goal of nursing care is to make patients feel accepted and respected while providing health care. This respect is demonstrated by both verbal and nonverbal communication. For example, some patients have difficulty maintaining personal hygiene or perhaps have a history of unhealthy behaviors such as smoking with a resulting diagnosis of lung cancer. Often, patients who have smoked are very aware of the impact of smoking on their health and bear some guilt or shame associated with these behaviors. The nurse's goal is to respectfully take into account the patient's symptoms, needs, values, and beliefs and collaborate to make decisions that are in his or her best interests. Oncology nurses demonstrate unconditional positive regard by accepting their patients without negatively judging their basic worth.

Veracity (Truth Telling)

Sharing the truth is never more apparent than when discussing communication behaviors between patients and healthcare providers. Oncology nurses are bound by codes of ethics to be honest with patients (ANA, 2015; International Council of Nurses, 2012). In addition, they are directed to promote ethical conduct by all healthcare providers, including reporting of unethical conduct. Sharing information with patients is crucial to helping them make decisions and adapt to changes in their health and treatment. However, truthfulness is more than the communication of facts; it also encompasses how information is communicated. In the 1950s and 1960s, doctors decided what information would be best for patients to know and believed that patients could maintain hope. This was a more paternalistic view of doctors protecting patients for their own benefit, or what doctors defined as "in the best interests" of patients. Doctors at that time often withheld information from patients. A doctor might have determined that telling a patient with breast cancer that she had metastatic disease and a limited life expectancy might be too upsetting and would remove her will to live. Now, patients in many Western countries desire and expect full disclosure of healthcare information and, sometimes, open access to all medical records. However, other cultures have varying approaches to sharing information. In some Arabic cultures, for example, families prefer that elders in the family make decisions about what information will be shared with the patient. Therefore, truth telling is more complex and requires balancing the characteristics of the patient, culture, and situation.

Self-Determination and Autonomy

The nursing profession has traditionally believed in the worth and dignity of all people seeking health care. The ethical principle of self-determination, or autonomy, guides nursing care and is the basis for informed decision making. Self-determination has roots in the ethical tradition of respect for persons. Patients have the right to determine what will and will not be done to, for, or with them. Nurses also demonstrate respect for persons by helping patients remain autonomous.

Patients have a range of expectations for their healthcare providers about sharing power and control, especially during times of decision making. Talking with patients often has been considered a central component of nursing practice. What is most important to patients is being treated in a friendly and respectful manner, being fully informed, and being given adequate consultation time (Moore, 2008). Nurses and patients have expectations about the nature of communication during interactions requiring assessment and clarification of the roles and needs of both parties. Although nurses often set the agenda for a visit ("Today, we will check your vital signs and blood counts and give you the second cycle of chemotherapy"), patients may have other concerns or expectations for the visit ("I need to talk with the social worker about my insurance because I do not know how I can pay for this chemotherapy"). Nurses can be clear about their role and agenda for a scheduled visit, but they also must assess the patient's needs to share control and decision making during the visit.

Advance directives are another example of patients' rights to self-determination about their health care. Decisions such as do-not-resuscitate orders and documents for durable power of attorney are examples of advance care directives that are completed by patients prior to circumstances that could limit their ability to make these choices or make these choices known.

The American Hospital Association first published *A Patient's Bill of Rights* in 1973 (revised in 1992 and replaced in 2003 by *The Patient Care Partnership* publication) to promote the rights of patients in the United States. Although many of these rights appear to be obvious, they were never formally adopted or distributed until the 1970s. Today, many insurance companies and health maintenance organizations also offer bills of rights to their patients. The Health Insurance Portability and Accountability Act (HIPAA Privacy Rule) of 1996 set national standards regarding the privacy of certain health information to protect people who seek care in the healthcare system. The compliance of healthcare providers or settings with HIPAA regulations often is defined in handouts that are provided to all patients. The same themes emerge in these documents about communication with patients that have roots in the ethical traditions of respect, autonomy, and privacy.

Values

Moral reasoning and decision making require the ability to examine both the nurse's values and the patient's values. Each nurse has a personal history and values that are brought to professional encounters with patients. Some values come from one's cultural and ethnic backgrounds, whereas others are accumulated over a lifetime of personal experiences that have shaped beliefs, attitudes, and communication styles. It is essential that nurses reflect on their values so they can identify and respect their patients' values even if they differ from their own. Without this reflection, unexplored values may become judgments and be expressed in communication or lack of communication with patients.

Values are formed from a person's beliefs about the truth, beauty, and worth of any thought, object, or behavior. They give direction and meaning to life and guide the decision-making process. Values also determine behavior and are one component in the generation of responses to complex ethical situations that arise in health care. Each nurse has values that may not be the same as the patients'. By separating patients' values from the nurses' values, nurses are better able to provide patient-centered care, care that respects patients' abilities (autonomy) to make choices about their health care. For example, a patient with a history of substance abuse develops a head and neck cancer requiring rigorous combined therapies. The nurse may acknowledge that he does not approve of the patient's history of substance abuse, but this judgment should not need to be communicated during care unless it affects the patient's response to treatment or affects symptom management. However, the facts about substance abuse may be part of a discussion about healthy behaviors in a nonjudgmental conversation. Nurses who develop awareness about their own values are better able to provide care that is respectful to patients.

Standards to Guide Communication

Nursing communication is guided by important rules and standards including patients' rights, professional standards, institutional standards, and legal statutes. During the 1960s, national leaders urged the healthcare system to become more responsive to patients' rights and needs. In addition, the public wanted to improve the quality of health care and hold healthcare providers and institutions accountable for the outcomes of care. Today, patients are assuming more responsibility for their own health, including adopting preventive health behaviors and following screening guidelines. Healthcare providers, such as oncology nurses, share in the responsibility to promote primary prevention (e.g., healthy eating, exercise) and screening tests (e.g., mammography, colonoscopy). Working with healthcare organizations, they can educate both patients and communities about the benefits of prevention and screening as well as early detection, diagnosis, and treatment of cancer.

Professional Standards

As healthcare professionals, nurses are required to adhere to the scope of their knowledge and practice. Central to nursing practice is respect for persons (ANA, 2015). For more than four decades, ANA has written and modified its *Code of Ethics for Nurses* to define the nursing role. The *Code of Ethics for Nurses* details the role of nurses, including their primary commitment to patients and their role as advocates for the health, safety, and rights of all patients. ANA also published *Nursing's Social Policy Statement: The Essence of the Profession* (2010), which defined nursing's value to society and the scope and standards of practice. These important public documents not only define the scope of nursing practice and the expected level of performance of nursing care but are also the standards by which nurses are held accountable by the judicial system. Additionally, these national documents are the basis for individual state nurse practice acts, the legal documents approved by each state's legislature that define the scope of nursing practice, nurses' rights and responsibilities, and licensure requirements. The scope of practice refers to legal and ethical parameters of nursing practice, including direct care, coordination of care with other disciplines including medicine and social work, and delegation of care to other personnel (such as certified nursing assistants). In the United States, a board of nursing oversees nursing practice in each state.

Patient Confidentiality

Patient confidentiality is an important issue from professional, legal, and institutional points of view. Confidentiality stems from the ethical tradition of a right to privacy. In addition, violating patient confidentiality is a breach of trust, which is an ethical component of patient care. As discussed previously, standards from the Office for Civil Rights and HIPAA define the protection of patients' individually identifiable data arising from encounters with healthcare services. Only information that is pertinent to patients' care can be shared with other providers who are directly involved in their care. For example, if a patient with cancer is receiving chemotherapy for lymphoma, this information cannot be shared with the patient's dentist unless the patient has given written permission.

Communication between a nurse and patient is considered to be privileged communication. This means that nurses are forbidden from disclosing information shared during nurse–patient interactions, with few exceptions. Legally, the nurse must disclose information to the appropriate authorities if the communication includes evidence that could harm innocent people, including the patient himself or herself. Other information that needs to be shared with authorities includes instances of child abuse, domestic abuse, gunshot wounds, and some communicable diseases, depending on the state.

Legal Standards

Laws define the boundaries and expectations of citizens to protect society and also define nursing practice. Legal statutes serve to protect the public and set standards for what constitutes professional nursing care. Based on tort law, the legal standard of a *reasonable standard of care* defines care that a reasonably prudent nurse would provide in a similar situation and also is used as a benchmark in courts of law to judge criminal negligence. It holds nurses accountable for their actions or their failure to act, such as failing to protect a patient from harm, performing a nursing action that a reasonably prudent nurse would not perform, or failing to perform an action that a reasonably prudent nurse would perform. For example, if a nurse hears a patient talking about methods to kill himself and does nothing to protect the patient from himself, then this is criminally negligent behavior. Unprofessional conduct related to communication may include breaching patient confidentiality, verbally abusing a patient, and falsifying records.

Communication Issues That Raise Ethical Dilemmas

Sensory Barriers

Barriers to communication may affect a patient's ability to communicate with nurses and other healthcare providers. Barriers may include the patient's ability to receive or express information that will impact his or her ability to understand the information and autonomously make decisions. Oncology nurses, by virtue of their time spent with patients, are in a unique position to identify and support patients' abilities and preferred methods of communication. In order to uphold ethical principles of respect, self-determination, and autonomy, nurses need to spend the extra time and effort to ensure that communication is just as effective with these patients as it is with patients who do not have sensory communication barriers. Nurses must work with an interprofessional healthcare team to facilitate services and make referrals to help patients communicate. When necessary, nurses also need to identify services or a support person or to act as a proxy to facilitate communication with and for patients who are unable to communicate effectively on their own.

Hearing Loss

Hearing loss can affect a patient's ability to receive information. For example, children with brain tumors may have hearing or speech deficits that require other methods of communication. Although parents are often good sources of information about their children, other methods such as sign language, word and picture boards, or hearing aids may facilitate communication. Older adult patients may have difficulty hearing because of age-related loss. Hearing aids are helpful in amplifying sound and eliminating background noise but may be difficult to maneuver and keep in place while in the hospital, resulting in patients not wearing them (Foust, 2014). Other times, older patients with hearing loss may choose not to use their hearing aids because the aids amplify too many sounds. Nurses can help patients by identifying hearing loss and employing adaptive equipment and devices or other methods to relay information to patients. Speaking in a loud voice may be a strategy that enhances communication with patients who have hearing loss, but it compromises patient privacy and confidentiality and should be used carefully with this consideration in mind.

Vision Loss

Vision loss may affect a patient's ability to read information, pick up on non-verbal cues, or assess surroundings. Vision changes may be because of aging, disease, or treatment. It is important that oncology nurses assess for visual changes including the type of loss (e.g., light, shadows, complete), medical condition (e.g., brain tumor, cataracts, glaucoma), and aids used and needed in the healthcare setting (e.g., braille, large print, glasses) (Foust, 2014). The use of aids should be incorporated into the care plan so that patients can maintain their usual functioning and adapted abilities while receiving health care, especially in acute care settings. For example, written information such as informed consent documents may be contraindicated if the patient has severe vision loss. Information may need to be relayed verbally, with opportunities for the patient to reflect understanding and ask questions to ensure effectiveness in sending, receiving, and assessing information.

Speech Loss

Language is the basic way of communicating with the world, both in receiving information and in conveying one's needs and feelings to others. Speech and language deficits may occur as part of the developmental or aging process or as a result of illness and treatment. Deficits may exist in receiving or expressing information and concerns. These deficits might last for brief periods of time, such as during intubation for mechanical ventilation, or they may result in permanent changes, such as after treatment for a brain tumor. For example, in the intensive care unit, a patient with leukemia may be sedated and ventilated as part of acute interventions to treat reversible conditions, such as neutropenic fever with pneumonia. The medical sedation may impair cognitive function, and the endotracheal tube may create aphasia. It is important to remember that patients will try to adapt to deficits, and nurses should use alternate methods to accommodate to these changes, such as picture boards, gestures, and writing tools. Nurses need to complete careful assessments and use tailored interventions to maximize patients' communication and autonomy (Foust, 2014).

Language Barriers

Communication can be particularly challenging when patients and nurses do not speak the same language. Even limited English proficiency can impact information gathering and decision making. In a comparative analysis of three international documents, five major ethical norms were identified as important for cross-linguistic nursing care: (a) respect for the patient as a unique person, (b) respect for the patient's right to self-determination, (c) respect for patient privacy and confidentiality, (d) responsibility for one's (the nurse's) own competence, judgment, and action, and (e) responsibility to promote action to more effectively meet the needs of vulnerable patients, families, and groups (Carnevale, Vissandjée, Nyland, & Vinet-Bonn, 2009).

Sometimes nurses use untrained interpreters such as family members, friends, and bilingual support staff to facilitate communication. However, there are often problems when family members and friends are used as interpreters, including their lack of familiarity with medical terminology in either language, deletion of important information because they cannot keep up, modification of meaning because they cannot make a literal translation, omission of pertinent sexual or sensitive information, and breach of confidentiality. These problems may lead to miscommunication and even serious medical errors (Rivadeneyra, Elderkin-Thompson, Silver, & Waitzkin, 2000).

Although family and friends are frequently convenient for translation, the use of trained interpreters improves the quality and safety of care delivery (Jacobs et al., 2001) and may even be mandated by legal statutes depending on the state. Trained interpreters have a higher degree of proficiency in both languages and medical terminology as well as special training in assistive strategies to improve communication. It is important that the nurse talks directly to the patient and has the interpreter stand behind the patient and to one side. This strategy promotes direct communication and respects patient autonomy. The nurse should ask the interpreter to translate directly and emphasize accuracy, completeness, and impartiality. When providing care to patients who require translation, nurses need to consider the extra time it may take to locate and schedule an interpreter and make these arrangements in advance whenever possible so that patient care is not delayed or postponed.

Communication of Bad News

Sharing bad news with patients is widely considered one of the most difficult aspects of patient–provider communication in cancer care. While oncologists most frequently have these discussions with patients, nurses are often present or consulted by patients and families before or after these conversations. When participating as part of the healthcare team in conversations with patients with advanced cancer, oncology nurses commonly encounter ethical dilemmas related to truth telling, family conflict, and offering treatments that might be considered futile (McLennon, Uhrich, Lasiter, Chamness, & Helft, 2013). Nurses must evaluate each situation carefully before intervening to share information about prognosis, treatment decisions, or advance care planning. If the nurse was not present for the conversation, it is best to know what was disclosed during the conversation with the oncologist prior to making decisions about further disclosure (Butts, 2013). Often more than one right decision can be made, thus requiring more discussion, time, and patience, with the focus remaining on the patient's right to choose.

Sharing bad news or making difficult treatment decisions may prompt strong emotional reactions in patients and families. While these are normal human responses, negative emotions may temporarily impair thinking and judgment. Working through these responses will help patients and families feel heard and respected, clearing the path for important decisions. Nurses and other healthcare providers are not immune to these strong responses, especially if they have formed long-standing relationships with patients. Negative emotions such as sadness, crying, and angry outbursts are not uncommon during difficult communication, but they may be uncomfortable for nurses to witness (Sheldon, Barrett, & Ellington, 2006).

Using the NURS pneumonic may be helpful in acknowledging patient emotions and providing respect and support (Fortin, Dwamena, Frankel, & Smith, 2012, pp. 21–22):

N—Name the emotion ("You sound upset today.")
U—Understand ("It has been a difficult day and this is understandable.")
R—Respect ("You have made it through tough times before.")
S—Support ("How can I help you?")

Most oncology nurses are not trained as therapists or mental health specialists, but they can use tools to help patients and families deal with strong emotions. Healthcare providers provide more empathic statements when speaking with patients who are expressing sadness and more medical information when speaking with patients who are expressing anger (Sheldon et al., 2009). Because expressions of anger may be signs of depression, frustration, or spiritual distress, it is important that nurses use tools such as the NURS pneumonic to help respond effectively to patients and families and provide the appropriate support or referral. The NURS pneumonic is also a useful tool for dealing with colleagues on the oncology team who may be experiencing moral distress during ethical dilemmas. Whatever the emotion, nurses must remember that ethical situations often arise because of conflict: conflict between people or even conflicting emotions within an individual. Conflict may give rise to anger, an emotion that is uncomfortable for many people, including oncology care providers. By acknowledging the heavy emotional load that often accompanies ethical situations, nurses can be supportive to their colleagues and team members and better communicate with patients and families.

Communication, Errors, and Malpractice

Patients have a right to quality and safe health care. Nursing, like medicine, is bound by the ethical obligation *to do no harm* to patients. Nurses play a critical role in ensuring that every patient has a safe encounter with healthcare providers at every visit. However, errors do occur, and many of these errors might have been prevented by better communication. In a 2004 report from the Joint Commission, 66% of sentinel events—errors or near errors with risk that resulted or could have resulted in critical injury or death—were caused by ineffective communication (Joint Commission, 2004). Given the frequency of communication errors, it is important to address how communication between patients and providers and within interdisciplinary teams has ethical implications for the delivery of safe health care.

Clear communication between patients and healthcare providers can prevent errors and decrease the incidence of malpractice claims. When huddles are done at the bedside, the patient should be included as a key informant about information and be involved in making decisions about care. Increasing patient assertiveness and requesting and respecting patient input may also be a more ethical approach to making decisions about care. This also demonstrates the ethical principles of *respect for persons* and *self-determination*. (See the Moral Map, developed by the Department of General Practice/Medical Ethics of the Academic Medical Center, Amsterdam, at www.moralmap.com for exercises on patient assertiveness.)

Even nurses with excellent clinical and communication skills may encounter patients who are dissatisfied with their care. In addition, nurses, like doctors and other healthcare providers, can be named in lawsuits. One of the best ways to decrease the incidence of dissatisfied patients and lawsuits is good communication between patients and healthcare providers. In a landmark study, patients who felt they were treated with respect and compassion sued healthcare providers less frequently (Levinson, Roter, Mullooly, Dull, & Frankel, 1997). Patients who feel that their providers really listen to them may be more satisfied with their care. It is important to remember that having a good "bedside manner" is not just being a nurse. Good communication skills increase the accuracy of assessments, create effective interventions, prevent complications, improve decision-making processes, and produce more satisfied patients. The same basic concepts of good communication—respect, empathy, and genuineness—may also prevent malpractice claims.

Oncology nurses advocate for patients within interdisciplinary teams. Their colleagues may include a variety of professionals such as oncologists, social workers, psycho-oncologists, nutritionists, physical therapists, and chaplains. Teamwork requires effective communication among team members to provide coordinated care and clear messages to patients and families. When effective, communication among team members facilitates the sharing of patient information, guides decision making, highlights areas of risk and need, and improves the efficacy of care delivery. For example, team huddles or rounds are increasingly being done at the bedside to share patient information, facilitate communication across disciplines, and develop care plans for patients. Lack of communication among team members may lead to fractured care, treatment delays, or even medical errors. Oncology nurses need to advocate for the nurse's voice on interdisciplinary oncology teams to facilitate information sharing and improve patient care delivery. Without teamwork, miscommunication may leave patients and families confused by inconsistent messages.

Team communication skills are necessary to ensure that information is shared among team members and relayed consistently to patients and families. Complex cases also require nurses to carefully navigate the healthcare system, advocating for patients and families by promoting effective communication between the team and the patient and family. Team communication may become strained during complex cases that involve ethical dilemmas, conflict, and strong emotions. The healthcare professions have collaborated to develop competencies to guide interprofessional communication. The Interprofessional Education Collaborative Expert Panel (2011) has specified four domains of interprofessional collaborative practice with related core competencies: (a) values and ethics, (b) roles and responsibilities, (c) communication, and (d) teamwork. These competencies echo important aspects of nurse communication on oncology teams and guide efforts and programs to improve communication with colleagues. Some communication tools for interprofessional teams include daily huddles, weekly patient safety meetings, multidisciplinary rounding, and rapid response teams.

In addition to communicating with patients and families and team members about patient care issues, oncology nurses are expected to participate in evaluation activities with team members. This communication may include giving feedback about a colleague's job performance or an organization's culture or responding appropriately when receiving feedback from others. Learning to give and receive timely, sensitive, and instructive feedback helps healthcare professionals improve the outcomes of team-based care. When a nurse is a member of an oncology team, constructive criticism is a valued component of team building, and patient safety and quality are the priority outcomes (Mulready-Shick & Foust, 2014).

A continuing education program that promotes excellence in communication in healthcare systems is TeamSTEPPS®, developed by the Agency for Healthcare Research and Quality (n.d.) and the Department of Defense to improve communication and teamwork regarding patient safety. TeamSTEPPS offers training curriculum packages tailored to diverse health systems that include multimedia modules and strategies for assessment, implementation, and sustainment of changes needed to create a culture of teamwork and effective communication. Included in these recommendations are using layman's terminology when speaking with patients and families to improve clarity and using standard language and terminology when speaking with team members. TeamSTEPPS also recommends verifying that the information received was the intended message of the sender. As discussed previously, this is a vital step in effective communication but one that is often overlooked during critical moments or intense discussions. Checking that the receiver heard information correctly and as intended by the sender is a crucial link in ensuring that communication took place.

During ethical dilemmas, nurses and oncologists have to negotiate multiple issues. For example, they may be caring for a patient who wishes to not undergo more treatment, while the patient's spouse requests more treatment, while simultaneously managing the realities of the diagnosis and prognosis. In one study of oncology nurses' perceptions of ethical dilemmas, nurses cited a need for more role clarification and interprofessional education about prognosis-related discussions (McLennon et al., 2013). Oncology team members must provide consistent messages when working through such ethical dilemmas. This may require a team huddle before meeting with a patient and his or her spouse to prevent miscommunication.

Electronic Health Communication

Increasingly, health information is shared between patients and providers via electronic means. These means include online sources of healthcare information, electronic and text prompts with health messages, and emails regarding health problems, questions, or even treatment (Weaver, Lindsay, & Gitelman, 2012). Electronic health record (EHR) systems also have electronic communication built into them, allowing providers to communicate with one another as part of administering an individual patient's care. When providers are using electronic health communication, concerns may arise over principles of confidentiality and privacy, as the ease of electronic communication may increase the risk of unauthorized access, sharing, and use of patient data. These concerns about security may inhibit some patients from reporting sensitive health data, which may compromise the validity of the patient record (Layman, 2008).

With email communication, concern exists for confidentiality and inclusion of the email into the EHR system as part of the permanent medical record. If the email is about a patient or with a patient, special care must be taken to ensure that the email is secure or encrypted and includes a disclaimer focusing on confidentiality and privacy laws warning the recipient of potential ramifications of the email being received by unintended parties. In addition to understanding the legal ramifications, a healthcare agency must make decisions and establish policies regarding the use of email and patient records. Similar to phone calls, email is void of the face-to-face contact that is so important in making complete clinical assessments. Although subjective data may be obtained, objective data may be lost. To communicate accurately, especially during complex situations with ethical considerations, face-to-face communication may be the best way to share information.

The use of electronic communication also raises issues related to justice and health disparities, as some socially disadvantaged patients may not have the same access to computerized communication as other patients. Electronic technologies such as the Internet are used more frequently by those who are more educated and have higher incomes, as well as patients who are younger (Viswanath, 2006). Therefore, healthcare professionals must assess the availability of computers or electronic devices for all patients and offer alternate modes of communication in cases where electronic communication is not feasible.

Culture and Communication

Culture is perceived as "the learned and shared behavior of a community of interacting human beings" (Useem, Useem, & Donoghue, 1963, p. 169). Lederach (1995) defined culture as the shared knowledge and schemes created by a set of people for perceiving, interpreting, expressing, and responding to the social norms around them. Several cultures have been identified in the United States today, each with its own set of unique standards that shape values and beliefs. Often, these beliefs differ from each other or from the norm of a community, demonstrating differences in views and thinking.

Particularly in the United States, many cultures differ from Western American culture. These cultural norms often shape the social and political values of individuals from a different culture, including their healthcare practices (Flammia, 2012; Purnell & Paulanka, 2008). To support a global community, moving away from an ethnocentric perspective is more effective (Flammia, 2012). Ethnocentrism, the belief that one's own culture is more dominant than other cultures, can be problematic because people who share this perspective tend to judge the behaviors of others in comparison to their own (Klopf, 1995). Cultural awareness stresses a drive away from ethnocentric views and focuses on understanding that individuals come from varying cultural background that influence how they interpret the world and relate to one another (Betancourt, Green, Carillo, & Ananeh-Firempong, 2003).

Cultural awareness is a key component in effective communication. Effective communication is accomplished when one person clearly understands the meaning and intention of what another person has said. Therefore, to effectively communicate, people must be culturally aware of values and norms of individuals of different cultures. In health care, this phenomenon is even more important because effective communication can influence informed decision making. Effective communication between healthcare professionals and patients generates information that is beneficial to patient outcomes and supports patient-centered care. Furthermore, it leads to increased patient knowledge and shared understanding, increased adherence to treatment recommendations, and adoption of healthier habits and self-care strategies (Epstein & Street, 2007).

Lack of cultural awareness can affect the quality and safety of nursing care. For example, Haitian immigrants have a range of religious beliefs and misconceptions about Western medicine (Stepick, 1998). Beyond language barriers, these beliefs and misconceptions can pose barriers to preventive medicine, including cancer screening (Green, Freund, Posner, & David, 2005; Kleier, 2009; Meade, Menard, Thervil, & Rivera, 2009; Menard et al., 2010). Religious and cultural beliefs are cherished in the Haitian culture and are perceived as the only constant, non-changing aspects of life (Purnell & Paulanka, 2008). Therefore, with the presentation of an illness, Haitians often turn to God in prayer as a religious practice and may use herbal medicine as a cultural practice to promote healing. Healthcare professionals must understand these beliefs when communicating with Haitian immigrants because often these traditional practices and views may be more influential in decision making and counteract with Western medicine recommendations. Acknowledging these beliefs can encourage a different approach to effective communication.

Intercultural communication promotes a feeling of being understood, supported, and respected in the individual with whom one is communicating (Ting-Toomey, 1999). This can be challenging, as Walsh (2014) reported, because high-context cultures tend to be indirect, where intuition and contemplation are valued more than reason and logic, and low-context cultures tend to be more direct, where words are important. Therefore, challenges may arise with communication between the two cultures because the needs and expectations are different. On one hand, healthcare professionals must treat patients and families fairly, and on the other hand, they must recognize what is efficient and most beneficial.

In becoming an intercultural communicator and taking into account ethical values, healthcare professionals should consider two philosophical concepts: universalism and cultural relativism. Universalism focuses on the belief that some ethical standards apply universally to all cultures (e.g., not causing harm to any patient). Cultural relativism argues that an individual from another culture cannot deem a behavior inappropriate. Thus, healthcare professionals must accept the decisions and beliefs of an individual from a different culture and seek ways to help influence interventions that may help improve health outcomes. Furthermore, Leininger (1978) proposed that healthcare professionals should respect patients' health beliefs and recognize their role in effective health care. Healthcare professionals should first listen to a patient's perception of illness or diagnosis and then share their perception of the illness and diagnosis (Leininger, 1978, 2002). Listening and sharing of information lead to effective communication that further leads to a desirable outcome for both parties involved.

No nurse will ever be an expert in the norms and beliefs of the various patient cultures, and to say that every individual in a particular culture is the same is not accurate. Familiarity with all cultural perspectives is not feasible, and viewing each patient as part of a particular group or culture can lead to stereotypes. Stereotyping may impact the quality of care and has been identified as a factor that contributes to persistent health disparities—that is, differences in the type of health care received and health outcomes achieved among diverse groups of people (Smedley, Stith, & Nelson, 2002).

Cultural awareness focuses on acquiring background knowledge about a particular culture and acknowledging the differences of that culture when compared to the majority (Saha, Beach, & Cooper, 2008). Being culturally competent and providing culturally competent care promote effective communication between patients and healthcare professionals and helps to eliminate healthcare disparities (Saha et al., 2008). To provide quality care, moving beyond one's own cultural perspective and understanding and acknowledging the norms of others are most important. Respecting others' beliefs and views minimizes judgment and promotes comfort for diverse individuals. Comfort promotes trust, and once comfortable, individuals are more likely to welcome interventions that may increase knowledge and encourage acceptance of Western medicine practices.

Implications for Nursing Practice

Oncology nurses have opportunities to create relationships with patients and families that improve outcomes of care. These relationships are particularly helpful when navigating difficult situations that have ethical implications. The effective use of communication skills with patients, families, and oncology team members can be very effective in promoting decision making with the patient's best interests. Oncology nurses send, receive, and assess communicated information to ensure the delivery and understanding of messages. They delve into their own values so as to be nonjudgmental in their care for patients. They advocate for patients' needs and values on the oncology team. Sometimes, as in the following case study, this means honoring the refusal of treatment (Hospice and Palliative Nurses Association, 2011). Oncology nurses communicate their willingness to work with patients and provide compassionate, sensitive, and knowledgeable care across the trajectory of care from diagnosis and survivorship to palliative and end-of-life care. Through effective communication, nurses identify patients' needs and values and advocate for their right to ethical, personal, and compassionate cancer care.

Case Study

When Melissa Nader arrives at the oncology department for her first consultation, she is 34 years old and newly diagnosed with stage III breast cancer. Pathologically, her tumor is estrogen and progesterone receptor positive and HER2/neu negative. She undergoes a mastectomy and reconstruction and then receives doxorubicin, cyclophosphamide, and paclitaxel in a dose-dense regimen followed by tamoxifen. Although her first scans do not show metastatic disease, within two years, Mrs. Nader develops liver and pulmonary metastases. Because of her young age, Mrs. Nader decides to enroll in a clinical trial for bevacizumab. During the trial, the lung nodules remain stable in size and her liver metastases shrink. Mrs. Nader tolerates her treatment well for 18 months until she develops disease progression. She is realistic and knows that she will never be cured of her disease but wants to live as long as possible for her young daughter, Megan.

During her six years of treatment, the oncology nurses develop a close relationship with Mrs. Nader and her family and understand her priorities. During this time, Mrs. Nader's marriage is a significant challenge to her quality of life. She and her husband, Rick, have been married for eight years. Rick is a first-generation Arab American who believes that men are the decision makers for the family. The couple's daughter is clearly the center of their world. Whenever Mrs. Nader is not feeling well, Mr. Nader becomes angry and controlling while Mrs. Nader remains even-tempered. Mr. Nader's angry outbursts become more frequent when her disease progresses. It is clear to the nurses that Rick's outbursts are stressful for Mrs. Nader, and they consult the social worker to provide support and counseling to Mrs. Nader as an individual and to them as a couple.

Unfortunately, two years after Mrs. Nader starts the clinical trial, her disease progresses with rapidly growing pulmonary metastases, and her performance status continues to decline each week. She quickly develops dyspnea with even mild exertion, experiences increased daytime sleepiness, and is sleeping in a recliner to lessen the work of breathing both at night and most of the day. One day, Mrs. Nader comes to the ambulatory oncology clinic with her husband. She is alert but has profound shortness of breath, tachycardia, and hypotension. The oncology team meets to discuss her case and how to handle the situation. Mrs. Nader had completed a do-not-resuscitate/do-not-intubate order one month ago but had not signed over durable power of attorney to her husband. She is admitted to the inpatient unit.

Mrs. Nader has an extensive workup to assess the extent of her disease, and the team concludes that she has developed left- and right-sided heart failure and is dying from her pulmonary metastases. The primary oncologist and nurse go to see Mrs. Nader in her room to discuss the test results. They find Mrs. Nader quiet in bed receiving nasal oxygen, gazing at the bedcover. Rick is pacing around the room, telling her that she "should not give up." He is furious that during the evening shift when he was home with their daughter, Mrs. Nader had chosen to have IV morphine for dyspnea. He wants more aggressive treatment, such as surgery to remove the pulmonary metastases and another regimen of chemotherapy. Mrs. Nader looks at her husband and then the oncology team and says, "No more. I know what this means. I am so tired and ready to go." The nurses are torn by Mrs. Nader's right to self-determination and become distressed when Rick yells about Mrs. Nader's "stupid decision." Mrs. Nader repeats her wishes again to her husband: "No more treatment. I know what this means, and I am all right with it. Can you make me go faster?"

The oncology nurse consults with the oncologist and the social worker about how to advocate for Mrs. Nader and also support Rick. It is clear to them that Mrs. Nader does not want any more treatment and is asking for ways to hasten the end of her life. The oncology nurse knows that they could honor Mrs. Nader's requests to withhold further treatment but they could not hasten her death (Hospice and Palliative Nurses Association, 2011). They discuss interventions to provide symptom management and relieve the suffering caused by the sense of breathlessness. Her husband is clearly distressed and needs reassurance and support so that he can support his wife during her last days.

First, the oncologist and nurse talk with Mrs. Nader and ask her permission to talk with Rick about the situation. Mrs. Nader is relieved and welcomes the help in talking with her husband, as she is "too tired." They have a frank discussion about treatment options and palliative care. Although Rick is hostile at first, he becomes silent and then tearful as they discuss the situation. He does not want his wife to die, but he expresses his desire for Mrs. Nader to be comfortable, to be with her, and for her to be able to see their daughter and family one more time. He comes to accept her desire for symptom relief with medications and her decision not to pursue further chemotherapy. The social worker then talks with Mrs. Nader and Rick about their needs for privacy and closure as Mrs. Nader approaches the end of her life. During the next few hours, the team gives Mrs. Nader and Rick some important time alone, while assuring them that the staff is close by to call if necessary.

Later that day, Mrs. Nader's mother brings Megan to visit. As requested by Rick, the nurse and social worker are present to help explain the situation in appropriate terms to the daughter as well as to Mrs. Nader's mother. Mrs. Nader removes the oxygen cannula, so as not to frighten Megan, and is able to cradle her daughter in her arms on the bed for more than an hour. Mrs. Nader dies a short time later with Rick at her side. Rick and Mrs. Nader's mother ask the oncology nurse to deliver words at Mrs. Nader's memorial service about her daughter's brave struggle against cancer and her willingness to talk honestly and openly about her cancer.

Discussion

This case study illustrates a difficult but not uncommon situation that can occur during end-of-life care in oncology settings. These situations often provoke strong responses and even moral distress in healthcare providers, especially if the providers have a long-term relationship with the patient (Ferrell & Coyle, 2008). Toward the end of her life, Mrs. Nader clearly communicated her preference not to have any more treatment. The nurse and team needed to support her wishes, even if they differed from her husband's wishes for surgery and more treatment. The interprofessional team worked together to develop a plan to support Mrs. Nader as well as each other. They held multiple discussions with her and her husband to provide information and make decisions about treatment options, approaches, and preferences. The team members also balanced the couple's need for privacy and intimate communication between themselves with being available to facilitate communication between the extended family.

Oncology nurses are often in the unique position to help patients and families with communication at the end of life. By nature of their professional goal to relieve suffering, nurses can help patients by listening to their concerns and understanding their physical and psychosocial symptom burden (Ferrell & Coyle, 2008). The nurses provided symptom management and supportive care to Mrs. Nader and her family. They advocated for Mrs. Nader and supported her right to self-determination. Mrs. Nader's husband also needed to have a supportive discussion with the oncology team to understand that his wife was dying and to deal with his strong emotions so that he could be more supportive to her and their daughter. The social worker, who had known the couple for several years, understood the cultural implications of Rick's responses as well as some of the dynamics within their marriage and family and was able to help them during this difficult time. She was able to be present during these important discussions and help the couple talk with their daughter. Mrs. Nader, with the help of the oncology nurse and team, was able to be present with her family, on her own terms, during the last part of her life.

Conclusion

Effective communication skills are an essential component of provident patient-centered care in oncology. When dealing with oncologic diagnoses, patients need healthcare professionals they can rely on and trust. Nurses are in a key position to fulfill part of that relationship. By understanding the basic concepts of communication and understanding the barriers to effective communication and how to overcome those barriers, nurses can not only be an advocate for patients through effective communication, but also can be a support to their interdisciplinary colleagues.

References

Agency for Healthcare Research and Quality. (2013). *TeamSTEPPS fundamentals course: Module 6—communication.* Retrieved from http://www.teamsteppsportal.org/component/phocadownload/category/47-module-6-communication

American Hospital Association. (2003). The patient care partnership. Retrieved from http://www.aha.org/advocacy-issues/communicatingpts/pt-care-partnership.shtml

American Nurses Association. (2010). *Nursing's social policy statement: The essence of the profession.* Retrieved from http://www.nursesbooks.org/Main-Menu/Foundation/Nursings-Social-Policy-Statement.aspx

American Nurses Association. (2015). *Code of ethics for nurses with interpretive statements.* Retrieved from http://www.nursingworld.org/DocumentVault/Ethics_1/Code-of-Ethics-for-Nurses.html

Betancourt, J.R., Green, A.R., Carrillo, J.E., & Ananeh-Firempong, O. (2003). Defining cultural competence: A practical framework for addressing racial/ethnic disparities in health and health care. *Public Health Reports, 118,* 293–302.

Butts, J.B. (2013). Ethics in professional nursing practice. In J.B. Butts & K.L. Rich (Eds.), *Nursing ethics: Across the curriculum and into practice* (3rd ed., pp. 69–98). Burlington, MA: Jones & Bartlett Learning.

Carnevale, F.A., Vissandjée, B., Nyland, A., & Vinet-Bonn, A. (2009). Ethical considerations in cross-linguistic nursing. *Nursing Ethics, 16,* 813–826. doi:10.1177/0969733009343622

Client. (n.d.). In *Merriam-Webster's collegiate dictionary* (11th ed.). Retrieved from http://www.merriam-webster.com/dictionary/client

Epstein, R.M., & Street, R.L., Jr. (2007). *Patient-centered communication in cancer care: Promoting healing and reducing suffering* [NIH Publication No. 07-6225]. Retrieved from https://pubs.cancer.gov/ncipl/detail.aspx?prodid=T099

Ferrell, B.R., & Coyle, N. (2008). The nature of suffering and the goals of nursing. *Oncology Nursing Forum, 35,* 241–247. doi:10.1188/08.ONF.241-247

Flammia, M. (2012). Preparing students for the ethical challenges of global citizenship. *Journal of Systemics, Cybernetics and Informatics, 10*(4), 41–45.

Fortin, A.H., Dwamena, F.C., Frankel, R.M., & Smith, R.C. (2012). *Smith's patient-centered interviewing: An evidence-based method* (3rd ed.). New York, NY: McGraw-Hill.

Foust, J.B. (2014). Physical impairments to communication. In L.K. Sheldon & J.B. Foust (Eds.), *Communication for nurses: Talking with patients* (3rd ed., pp. 131–150). Burlington, MA: Jones & Bartlett Learning.

Green, E.H., Freund, K.M., Pösner, M.A., & David, M.M. (2005). Pap smear rates among Haitian immigrant women in eastern Massachusetts. *Public Health Reports, 120,* 133–139.

Hospice and Palliative Nurses Association. (2011). Role of the nurse when hastened death is requested [Position statement]. Retrieved from http://hpna.advancingexpertcare.org/wp-content/uploads/2015/08/Role-of-the-Nurse-When-Hastened-Death-is-Requested.pdf

International Council of Nurses. (2012). *The ICN code of ethics for nurses.* Retrieved from http://www.icn.ch/images/stories/documents/about/icncode_english.pdf

Interprofessional Education Collaborative Expert Panel. (2011). *Core competencies for interprofessional collaborative practice: Report of an expert panel.* Washington, DC: Author.

Jacobs, E.A., Lauderdale, D.S., Meltzer, D., Shorey, J.M., Levinson, W., & Thisted, R.A. (2001). Impact of interpreter services on delivery of health care to limited-English-proficient patients. *Journal of General Internal Medicine, 16,* 468–474. doi:10.1046/j.1525-1497.2001.016007468.x

Joint Commission. (2004). Sentinel event alert. Retrieved from http://www.jointcommission.org/assets/1/18/sea_30.pdf

Kleier, J.A. (2009). Language adaptation and psychometric estimation of measures of fear of and susceptibility to prostate cancer among Haitian-American men. *Urologic Nursing, 29,* 425–433.

Klopf, D.W. (1995). *Intercultural encounters: The fundamentals of intercultural communication* (3rd ed.). Englewood, CO: Morton.

Layman, E.J. (2008). Ethical issues and the electronic health record. *Health Care Manager, 27,* 165–176.

Lederach, J.P. (1995). *Preparing for peace: Conflict transformation across cultures.* Syracuse, NY: Syracuse University Press.

Leininger, M. (1978). *Transcultural nursing: Concepts, theories, and practices.* New York, NY: Wiley.

Leininger, M. (2002). Essential transcultural nursing care concepts, principles, examples, and policy statements. In M. Leininger & M.R. McFarland (Eds.), *Transcultural nursing: Concepts, theories, research and practice* (3rd ed., pp. 45–69). New York, NY: McGraw-Hill.

Levinson, W., Roter, D.L., Mullooly, J.P., Dull, V.T., & Frankel, R.M. (1997). Physician-patient communication: The relationship with malpractice claims among primary care physicians and surgeons. *JAMA, 277,* 553–559. doi:10.1001/jama.1997.03540310051034

McIntyre, R.M., & Salas, E. (1995). Measuring and managing for team performance: Lessons from complex environments. In R.A. Guzzo, E. Salas, & Associates (Eds.), *Team effectiveness and decision making in organizations* (pp. 9–45). San Francisco, CA: Jossey-Bass.

McLennon, S.M., Uhrich, M., Lasiter, S., Chamness, A.R., & Helft, P.R. (2013). Oncology nurses' narratives about ethical dilemmas and prognosis-related communication in advanced cancer patients. *Cancer Nursing, 36,* 114–121. doi:10.1097/NCC.0b013e31825f4dc8

Meade, C.D., Menard, J., Thervil, C., & Rivera, M. (2009). Addressing cancer disparities through community engagement: Improving breast health among Haitian women. *Oncology Nursing Forum, 36,* 716–722. doi:10.1188/09.ONF.716-722

Menard, J., Kobetz, E., Maldonado, J.C., Barton, B., Blanco, J., & Diem, J. (2010). Barriers to cervical cancer screening among Haitian immigrant women in Little Haiti, Miami. *Journal of Cancer Education, 25,* 602–608. doi:10.1007/s13187-010-0089-7

Moore, M. (2008). What does patient-centred communication mean in Nepal? *Medical Education, 42,* 18–26. doi:10.1111/j.1365-2923.2007.02900.x

Mulready-Shick, J., & Foust, J.B. (2014). Practicing conflict resolution, negotiation, and interprofessional and intraprofessional collaboration. In L.K. Sheldon & J.B. Foust (Eds.), *Communication for nurses: Talking with patients* (3rd ed., pp. 229–246). Burlington, MA: Jones & Bartlett Learning.

National Commission for the Protection of Human Subjects of Biomedical and Behavioral Research. (1979, April 18). *The Belmont Report: Ethical principles and guidelines for the protection of human subjects of research.* Retrieved from http://www.hhs.gov/ohrp/humansubjects/guidance/belmont.html

Patient. (n.d.). In *Merriam-Webster's collegiate dictionary* (11th ed.). Retrieved from http://www.merriam-webster.com/dictionary/patient

Peplau, H.E. (1952). *Interpersonal relations in nursing.* New York, NY: Putnam.

Peplau, H.E. (1992). Interpersonal relations: A theoretical framework for application in nursing practice. *Nursing Science Quarterly, 5,* 13–18. doi:10.1177/089431849200500106

Purnell, L.D., & Paulanka, B.J. (2014). *Transcultural health care: A culturally competent approach* (2nd ed.). Philadelphia, PA: F.A. Davis.

Rivadeneyra, R., Elderkin-Thompson, V., Silver, R.C., & Waitzkin, H. (2000). Patient centeredness in medical encounters requiring an interpreter. *American Journal of Medicine, 108,* 470–474. doi:10.1016/S0002-9343(99)00445-3

Rogers, C.R. (1961). *On becoming a person: A therapist's view of psychotherapy.* Boston, MA: Houghton Mifflin.

Saha, S., Beach, M.C., & Cooper, L.A. (2008). Patient centeredness, cultural competence and healthcare quality. *Journal of the National Medical Association, 100,* 1275–1285.

Sheldon, L.K., Barrett, R., & Ellington, L. (2006). Difficult communication in nursing. *Journal of Nursing Scholarship, 38,* 141–147. doi:10.1111/j.1547-5069.2006.00091.x

Sheldon, L.K., Ellington, L., Barrett, R., Clayton, M.F., Dudley, W.N., & Rinaldi, K. (2009). Nurse responsiveness to cancer patient expressions of emotion. *Patient Education and Counseling, 76,* 63–70. doi:10.1016/j.pec.2008.11.010

Smedley, B.D., Stith, A.Y., & Nelson, A.R. (Eds.). (2002). *Unequal treatment: Confronting racial and ethnic disparities in health care.* Washington, DC: National Academies Press.

Stepick, A. (1998). *Pride against prejudice: Haitians in the United States.* Boston, MA: Allyn & Bacon.

Ting-Toomey, S. (1999). *Communicating across cultures.* New York, NY: Guilford Press.

Useem, J., Useem, R., & Donoghue, J. (1963). Men in the middle of the third culture: The roles of American and non-Western people in cross-cultural administration. *Human Organization, 22,* 169–179.

Viswanath, K. (2006). Public communications and its role in reducing and eliminating health disparities. In G.E. Thomson, F. Mitchell, & M.B. Williams (Eds.), *Examining the health disparities research plan of the National Institutes of Health: Unfinished business* (pp. 215–253). Washington, DC: Institute of Medicine.

Walsh, J.H. (2014). Cross-cultural communication. In L.K. Sheldon & J.B. Foust (Eds.), *Communication for nurses: Talking with patients* (3rd ed., pp. 41–58). Burlington, MA: Jones & Bartlett Learning.

Weaver, B., Lindsay, B., & Gitelman, B. (2012). Communication technology and social media: Opportunities and implications for healthcare systems. *Online Journal of Issues in Nursing, 17*(3), 3. Retrieved from http://nursingworld.org/MainMenuCategories/ANAMarketplace/ANAPeriodicals/OJIN

CHAPTER 7

Genetics and Genomics

Dale Halsey Lea, MPH, RN, CGC

Introduction

Genetics and genomics are becoming an essential component of nursing practice, including oncology, as nearly all diseases and health conditions have a genetic or genomic component. Genetic testing and technologies are being used for the prevention, screening, diagnosis, and treatment of both rare and common diseases. Oncology nurses will increasingly be involved in providing genomic-based health care and translating new genetic and genomic information to patients and their families while keeping in mind associated ethical issues of importance (Lea, 2008). Having an understanding of the ethical, legal, and social issues related to genetic and genomic information and their translation into clinical practice is essential to the provision of safe, effective, and competent care to patients, families, and communities (Badzek, Henaghan, Turner, & Monsen, 2013). This chapter will address four important ethical issues related to genetics and genomics in health care that are key to oncology nurses' knowledge base: (a) informed consent, (b) privacy and confidentiality, (c) genetic discrimination, and (d) direct-to-consumer genetic testing. Approaches that oncology nurses can use to address ethical issues related to genetics and genomics in health care also will be discussed.

Overview

In 2003, the Human Genome Project, an international, collaborative research program, was completed. The overall goal of the Human Genome Project was to completely map and identify all of the genes in a human being. This included identifying the approximately 20,500 genes in a human being and determining the sequences of the three billion chemical base pairs that make up human DNA. All of the genes in a human being are now known as an individual's genome. The study of a particular gene is known as *genetics*, whereas the study of an entire genome of an organism, including gene interactions with each other, the environment, and the influence of other psychosocial and cultural factors, is referred to as *genomics* (National Human Genome Research Institute [NHGRI], 2014d). The results of the Human Genome Project have provided researchers with detailed information about the structure, function, and organization of all human genes that provide instructions for the development and function of each individual. Information and data gained from the Human Genome Project have been made available to researchers and others who are interested in the role of genetics in human health (NHGRI, 2012c).

A gene is defined as the basic functional and physical unit of heredity. A gene is made up of DNA that provides the instructions to create proteins. Individuals have two copies of each gene and inherit one from each parent. It is now known that most genes are similar in all people, and only less than 1% of genes differ among individuals. Each individual's unique physical features are the result of this small difference (Genetics Home Reference, 2014).

Genes are packaged into structures called *chromosomes*, which are located in the nucleus of cells. Human beings have 23 pairs of chromosomes: 22 of the pairs are called *autosomes*, and the 23rd pair is called *sex chromosomes*. Females have two X chromosomes, and males have one X chromosome and one Y chromosome. The complete set of chromosomes in an individual is known as a *karyotype* (Genetics Home Reference, 2014). The collection of genes in an individual is known as the *genotype*, and the expression of the genotype contributes to that person's observable physical traits. The physical manifestation of a person's genotype in the form of a trait such as eye color, height, or disease such as cancer is referred to as the *phenotype* (NHGRI, 2014f).

This expanding knowledge of the role of genes in health and disease is leading to a new era in health care called *personalized medicine*. Personalized medicine is a new practice that uses a person's genetic makeup to help determine methods to screen for, diagnose, and treat disease. Knowing a person's genetic profile, for example, is now beginning to help healthcare providers to choose the appropriate medication or treatment for particular conditions, such as breast cancer, and also to administer the drug using the appropriate dose (NHGRI, 2014e). As Francis S. Collins, MD, PhD, former director of NHGRI at the National Institutes of Health, noted about a person's genetic makeup, "It's a history book—a narrative of the journey of our species through time. It's a shop manual, with an incredibly detailed blueprint for building every human cell. And it's a transformative textbook of medicine, with insights that will give health care providers immense new powers to treat, prevent and cure disease" (NHGRI, 2012c, para. 6).

These advances in genetics and genomics have significant implications for individuals, families, and society in obtaining and possessing detailed genetic and genomic information. The Human Genome Project recognized these implications from the beginning and led genetic researchers to the ongoing analysis of the ethical, legal, and social implications of the newly discovered genetic information and knowledge and development of specific policy options for the public's consideration (NHGRI, 2012c).

Informed Consent

Informed consent involves a process to assist patients and usually their families and loved ones to understand the purpose and benefits of proposed treatment as well as its risks and benefits. Patients must be able to provide their consent without feeling coerced (NHGRI, 2012a), and an appropriate surrogate decision maker can consent on their behalf. As genetics and genomics are increasingly incorporated into health care, nurses will be more involved in the informed consent and decision-making processes. As noted in the *Essentials of Genetic and Genomic Nursing: Competencies, Curricula Guidelines, and Outcome Indicators,* nurses' professional responsibilities include advocating "for the rights of all clients for autonomous, informed genetic- and genomic-related decision-making and voluntary action" (Consensus Panel on Genetic/Genomic Nursing Competencies, 2009, p. 11).

Nurses who care for patients in primary and specialty care settings such as oncology will be increasingly involved in collecting and reviewing patients' family histories. An important nursing responsibility is to explain the reason and purpose for collecting family history before asking for and obtaining the patient's verbal consent. If the nurse is required to obtain family history from related family members, then he or she must support and protect the confidentiality of all family members by privately collecting the family history again from each of the other family members (Lea, 2008).

As the use of genetic testing expands throughout the life continuum in the areas of screening, diagnosis, and determining treatment for both rare and common diseases, nurses will become more involved in assisting patients throughout their decision-making and informed consent processes. They will help patients understand the reason for the genetic test as well as the risks and benefits. For example, oncology nurses now are involved in genetic testing for hereditary breast, ovarian, and other cancers. Nurses must have an understanding of the informed consent process. This process has been found to be most effective when it involves questions and answers between the patient and his or her practitioner and requires that the practitioner use an appropriate level of technical detail and language that is suitable for the patient's understanding (Athena Diagnostics, 2013). Nurses also may be involved in the process of obtaining a patient's written consent to share results of his or her genetic testing with other family members or to use a patient's biologic samples for research purposes (Lea, 2008).

An emerging ethical issue involved with informed consent and genetic testing involves the possible use of predictive genetic testing of children for an adult-onset disorder such as cancer. Genetic testing of children for adult-onset disorders excludes the child's right to informed choice and consent and puts the child at risk for discrimination and lifelong stigma (American Academy of Pediatrics Committee on Bioethics, 2001). In 2013, the American Academy of Pediatrics and the American College of Medical Genetics issued recommendations about genetic testing of children to guide healthcare providers on when it is appropriate to test a child's DNA for genetic conditions. They recommended that testing children for genetic diseases that do not affect individuals until adulthood, such as testing a young girl for *BRCA1* and *BRCA2* mutations associated with hereditary breast and ovarian cancer, should be discouraged unless a treatment is available that can reduce the child's risk of complications or death. However, the experts agreed that an exception to this recommendation can be made if the testing will relieve the parents' emotional burden of not knowing whether the child does or does not have a particular condition (American Academy of Pediatrics, 2013; Seaman, 2013).

Privacy and Confidentiality

As genetic technologies expand and are increasingly used in health care, new sources of medical information for individuals, families, and communities are raising important ethical, legal, and social issues. Nurses must be familiar with the nature and sources of genetic information so that they can ensure privacy and confidentiality for their patients (Lea, 2008). As a first step, nurses need to understand how genetic information is defined. Genetic information is both biologic and heritable.

Nurses also need to understand how privacy and confidentiality are defined. The American Nurses Association's (ANA's) *Code of Ethics for Nurses* defined privacy as a person's right to control his or her own personal information and access to and disclosure of this information. It also defined confidentiality as the nurse's obligation to protect and not disclose an individual's personal information that has been provided as part of the nurse–patient relationship (ANA, 2015). Nurses have a critical role in ensuring the privacy and confidentiality of their patients' genetic information. The International Society of Nurses in Genetics (ISONG) position statement on privacy and confidentiality of genetic information states that maintaining privacy and confidentiality of genetic information "demands continued vigilance on the part of all nurses as genetic technologies and discoveries are translated into clinical application and practice" (ISONG, 2010, p. 1).

An ethical dilemma can occur when genetic information gathered from genetic testing or family history reveals information about a patient's health risk that other family members may also be at risk for but are not aware of. Nurses face a conflict in that they are required to respect the patient's confidentiality and right to privacy of genetic information and yet have the responsibility to warn other family members of their possible health risks. For example, a male patient has a family history of Huntington disease (HD) in his father's family. His father died from HD. The patient decides to be tested to see if he has the gene that causes HD. He learns that he does have the HD gene and therefore will develop the disease. He has three children but has not been in touch with them since his divorce from their mother several years earlier. He tells the nurse that he does not want to share this information with his children because he feels it is none of their business. The concern for his children is that they now have a 1 in 2 (50%) risk of inheriting the HD gene that their father has. The nurse can find guidance in the *Code of Ethics for Nurses* (ANA, 2015), which recommends that the nurse reach out for assistance and counsel from experienced individuals on the ethics committee or another similar resource within the institution.

Nurses can best help a patient's family members by clearly informing patients who are identified as having a gene mutation that causes a genetic condition or test positive for a genetic condition about the risks that their family members face and talking with them about the importance and value of disclosing this genetic information (Gallo, Angst, & Knafl, 2009; International Council of Nurses, 2012). Nurses also should be aware of the Health Insurance Portability and Accountability Act (HIPAA) Privacy Rule, which provides federal protections for an individual's personal health information. HIPAA requires healthcare providers, as well as third-party payers and healthcare clearinghouses, to ensure protection of the privacy and security of health information, including genetic information, that could lead to identifying a person. It provides patients with their rights over their health information and includes rules and limits on who can view and receive their health information. Simultaneously, the HIPAA Privacy Rule also allows for the disclosure of personal health information that is needed for patient care and research (U.S. Department of Health and Human Services, n.d.).

Privacy and confidentiality issues also can arise in genetic research studies. For example, these issues may come up with genetic family studies because of the familial relationship between the family members participating in the research. It is important for those working in this area of genetic research to understand that each family member is an individual who deserves to have his or her information kept private and confidential. This means that other family members do not have the right to information about each other's diagnoses. Therefore, research investigators are obligated to obtain the consent of research participants before providing this medical or personal information to other family members (NHGRI, 2012d).

A type of genetic testing called *whole genome sequencing* soon will become available and offered to patients in clinics at the cost of approximately $1,000 per individual genome. This type of testing is very promising but also raises concerns about the privacy of a patient's whole genome sequencing information. For example, when a patient has this type of genetic testing, the information gained from the whole genome sequencing could have implications for other family members. In addition, unanticipated findings may come about over the years that follow after the whole genome sequencing test that may cause concerns. Concerns regarding maintaining privacy of this sensitive information about individual patients also have been raised. In recognition of these privacy concerns, President Barack Obama's Presidential Commission for the Study of Bioethical Issues developed a report titled *Privacy and Progress in Whole Genome Sequencing*. The report recognized that whole genome sequencing is promising and can help researchers in genetics and genomics identify genetic causes of rare and common diseases. However, the report also noted that large genome data collection could raise significant privacy concerns because of the risk that this important and sensitive medical information may not remain private. The report proposed that a balanced approach be taken when developing privacy policies, as it is possible that attempting to protect the privacy of genetic information may constrain research programs. The report also stressed the importance of informing patients about what it means to have their whole genome sequenced (Kaiser, 2012).

Genetic Discrimination

The Ethical, Legal and Social Implications Research Program at NHGRI recognized early on that discrimination based on an individual's genetic information was an important ethical issue to be addressed as the Human Genome Project moved forward (NHGRI, 2012c). Many individuals already were concerned that their personal genetic information showing that they had differences in their DNA that increased their chances of developing a certain disease would be misused and cause employment and insurance discrimination. This is known as *genetic discrimination*. For example, a health insurance company could decline coverage to a man who has DNA differences that increase his chances of developing colon cancer. Another instance of genetic discrimination could arise if an employer decides to use a person's DNA information to determine who to hire and which workers to fire (NHGRI, 2014b). As the use of genetic testing expands and becomes a routine part of health care, healthcare providers will increasingly use an individual's DNA information in screening, diagnosis, and treatment to individualize his or her health care. However, it was recognized that if the DNA information was not protected, it could lead to discrimination against individuals.

In recognizing the potential for discrimination based on a person's DNA information, the Genetic Information Nondiscrimination Act, also known as GINA, was created and signed into law in 2008 by President George W. Bush. GINA prevents employers and insurers from discriminating against individuals based on their DNA information. GINA also supports individuals' participation in research studies without being concerned that their genetic information could be used against them at work or by their health insurance company. However, GINA does not cover long-term care insurance, life insurance, or disability insurance (NHGRI, 2014c; U.S. Department of Health and Human Services, 2009).

Nurses in all practice settings, along with other healthcare providers, have the responsibility to protect patients and families from the misuse of their genetic information. As a part of their work with healthcare providers, nurses help with the creation of practice settings that provide patients with assurance that their personal genetic information will be shared in a professional manner (Consensus Panel on Genetic/Genomic Nursing Competencies, 2009). Therefore, nurses must become familiar with GINA and its provisions so they can assure their patients that there is now a federal law in place that protects the use of their personal genetic information in employment and health insurance decisions (Beery & Workman, 2012).

Direct-to-Consumer Genetic Testing

A number of different types of genetic tests are now being offered to consumers directly and do not involve healthcare providers in the process. These tests, called direct-to-consumer (DTC) genetic tests, instruct individuals to scrape cells from the inside of their cheek and then send the sample to the company that will perform the tests in their laboratory. Healthcare providers are usually not involved with the ordering of DTC genetic tests. One type of DTC genetic test is known as a *nutrigenetic test*, which provides information about an individual's genetic makeup that can be used to create an individualized diet plan. DTC genetic tests also can provide health-related information such as changes in all or parts of a person's genome that may affect his or her risk of developing a particular disease. DTC genetic tests also are used to identify genetic variants that may be related to certain aspects of an individual's life, such as physical traits or personality (NHGRI, 2014a).

One of the biggest concerns surrounding DTC genetic testing since it began is the accuracy of tests. The Government Accountability Office explored this issue in 2006 by submitting a number of samples from two sources with fictitious consumer profiles to four different websites that offered DTC genetic tests for diseases such as heart disease and cancer. The study revealed that the results were misleading because they provided predictions of diseases that were inconsistent for identical samples and used language that was ambiguous in describing results (NHGRI, 2012b).

The American Society of Human Genetics (ASHG) also issued a statement on DTC genetic testing in 2007, advising that consumers are at risk for harm if they use these tests (Hudson, Javitt, Burke, Byers, & ASHG Social Issues Committee, 2007). They recommended that health professional organizations educate their members about the types and nature of DTC genetic testing so that they can provide their patients with information about the potential risks and limitations of this type of genetic testing. They also recommended that relevant federal government agencies should take appropriate regulatory action to ensure that the DTC genetic tests are analytically and clinically valid (Hudson et al., 2007).

In 2009, ISONG developed a position statement on DTC genetic testing and important nursing roles. The statement outlined the identified risks of DTC genetic testing, including the delivery of genetic test results without the involvement of or advice from genetics professionals or healthcare providers. Without the guidance and advice of these healthcare professionals, individuals who have had DTC genetic testing may misinterpret the risks and fail to take appropriate preventive behaviors because the risks were not presented adequately. Furthermore, with all of the concerns about the accuracy of DTC genetic tests, nurses need to be responsible for promoting risk reduction by recommending that patients consult with genetics professionals to help them understand when genetic tests are appropriate and the concerns about DTC testing (ISONG, 2009).

Implications for Nursing Practice

Genetic and genomic technologies and information are having a significant impact on health and disease throughout an individual's life span. Therefore, healthcare providers in all areas of practice will be moving from the one-size-fits-all approach to individualized health care based on the patient's genetic and genomic profile. This new approach to screening, diagnosis, and treatment of rare and common diseases known as personalized medicine is opening the doors for all nurses to participate in more personalized health care at all stages throughout the life span and for all populations. This includes increasing participation in the genetic testing process, collecting family history, administering gene-based therapies and treatments, and creating genomic-based healthcare plans for patients (Lea, 2008).

In order for all nurses to participate fully in genomic-based personalized health care, they need to demonstrate that they are proficient in incorporating genetic and genomic information into their practice. An important element of nursing competency in genetics and genomics is knowledge and awareness of the current and emerging ethical issues in genomic health care. These include ensuring informed consent for genetic testing and treatment and maintaining privacy and confidentiality of a patient's genetic and genomic information in both clinical and research settings. Nurses must also ensure that patients are not discriminated against for job opportunities or health insurance based on their genetic and genomic information. Nurses need to be aware of new genetic tests marketed directly to patients and families without healthcare providers being involved and should be familiar with the accuracy and meaning of such genetic testing (Badzek et al., 2013).

To provide individualized and safe genomic health care, nurses first need to become aware of and examine their own ethical concerns and beliefs regarding genetics and genomics so that these beliefs will not interfere with supportive health care. *Essentials of Genetic and Genomic Nursing* recommended that as a first step all nurses need to "recognize when one's own attitudes and values related to genetic and genomic science may affect care provided to clients" (Consensus Panel on Genetic/Genomic Nursing Competencies, 2009, p. 11). Having knowledge of their attitudes and values regarding genetic and genomic ethical issues will support and ensure that nurses are able to provide higher quality and ethically based genetic and genomic nursing care for all patients, families, and communities (Lea, 2008).

Case Study

Women's Health: Part One

Jane Harris is a nurse working in a family practice healthcare clinic. One of her first patients of the day is Barbara Cohen, a 42-year-old woman who is at the clinic for her annual health checkup. This is her first visit to the clinic. One of Ms. Harris' duties as a nurse is to collect and record Mrs. Cohen's family history. Mrs. Cohen tells Ms. Harris that she has three sisters, ages 44, 46, and 48, who do not have any health problems. Mrs. Cohen has a 15-year-old daughter and a 17-year-old son, both of whom are in good health, as well as a husband in good health. She tells Ms. Harris that her mother was an only child and is now 72 and in good health. Her father is 74 and has a history of high blood pressure. He had one sister who died from ovarian cancer at age 44. His mother died at age 50 from breast cancer. His father died of a heart attack at age 88. Mrs. Cohen also tells Ms. Harris that both of her parents are of Ashkenazi Jewish ancestry and that she is worried about the history of breast and ovarian cancer in her father's family. She asks Ms. Harris if she could be at risk for breast or ovarian cancer even though the history is on her father's side. Ms. Harris tells Mrs. Cohen that it is a possibility and that she would like to refer her for genetic counseling for further evaluation of her family history.

Mrs. Cohen agrees to the genetic counseling. After receiving the counseling, she gets back in touch with Ms. Harris to set up an appointment. At the appointment, she tells Ms. Harris that the geneticist had informed her that early-onset breast and ovarian cancer can be inherited in families through maternal and paternal relatives. She was also told that individuals of Ashkenazi Jewish descent have a higher risk of hereditary breast and ovarian cancer because of mutations in the *BRCA1* and *BRCA2* genes. The geneticist tells her about genetic testing that is available to learn whether she carries one of the genes that could predispose her to breast and ovarian cancer. Mrs. Cohen states that she has decided to go forward with the genetic testing but will pay for it out of pocket because she does not want her insurance company to know about the results and discriminate against her if they are positive. How should Ms. Harris address Mrs. Cohen's concern about discrimination by her insurance company based on her genetic test results?

Discussion

As a nurse, Ms. Harris would know that GINA prevents employers and insurers from discriminating against individuals based on their DNA information. GINA also supports individuals' participation in research studies without fear that their genetic information could be used against them at work or by their health insurance company. Ms. Harris could inform Mrs. Cohen about GINA and assure her that this federal law protects against the use of her personal genetic information in health insurance and employment decisions.

Part Two

Mrs. Cohen's genetic test results show that she carries a mutation in the *BRCA1* gene, meaning that she is at increased risk for developing early-onset breast and/or ovarian cancer. At a follow-up visit, Mrs. Cohen tells Ms. Harris that the geneticist said that each of her sisters has a 50% risk for inheriting the same *BRCA1* mutation from their father. Mrs. Cohen also tells Ms. Harris that she does not get along with her sisters and has not spoken to them in years. She says that she does not want to tell them about her gene mutation. She states, "Let them find out for themselves. It is not my job to tell them." How should Ms. Harris respond to Mrs. Cohen's decision?

Discussion

To help patients and families make decisions about disclosing genetic risk information—and to avoid undue distress in the process—nurses must understand the many issues that may affect families, such as sharing genetic information with family members. Whether people like Mrs. Cohen who have a *BRCA1* gene mutation choose to disclose genetic information to family members may depend on how close they feel to those family members as well as their sense of responsibility to them. When patients decide not to disclose their genetic test results and risk of developing a genetic condition such as hereditary breast and ovarian cancer, this can pose a dilemma for nurses and healthcare professionals who must make a choice between their ethical obligations to inform at-risk family members and the legal requirements to respect and protect patient privacy.

In these situations, nurses and healthcare providers need to carefully explain the reasons it is important for patients to share the information with at-risk relatives and offer to help them develop a plan to inform them about the risk. If a patient chooses not to notify family members, healthcare providers usually respect this decision; however, in some situations a healthcare provider may consider overriding the patient's decision because the family members are thought to be at risk for serious or immediate harm, or when a condition can be prevented or treated adequately. When healthcare providers determine that they need to override a patient's decision to not notify at-risk family members, they should consider consulting an ethics committee or legal counsel. In situations like Mrs. Cohen's, where the risk of her sisters inheriting the *BRCA1* gene mutation is 50% and they do not have a 100% chance of developing breast or ovarian cancer if they inherit the gene, the need for disclosure is not as urgent as with more serious genetic disorders. In this situation, Ms. Harris must help Mrs. Cohen to learn more about the mutation and what it means for her and her children, as well as the risks faced by her sisters. Ms. Harris could help Mrs. Cohen to give careful thought on how and when she could share her test results with her sisters. Gallo et al. (2009) offered more information about ethical issues that may arise when disclosing genetic information to family members and how nurses can help families.

Mrs. Cohen's decision not to share her *BRCA1* results with her sisters poses a significant dilemma for Ms. Harris, who now has to choose between ethical obligations to inform Mrs. Cohen's at-risk sisters and her legal requirements to protect Mrs. Cohen's privacy. Ms. Harris decides to continue explaining to Mrs. Cohen the reasons that it is important for her to share her *BRCA1* information with her sisters. She continues to clearly inform Mrs. Cohen about the risks that her sisters face and explains the value of disclosure. Ms. Harris also offers to assist Mrs. Cohen with disclosing this information. After hearing this information from Ms. Harris, Mrs. Cohen tells Ms. Harris that she has decided to inform her sisters that about her *BRCA1* results and their potential risk to have inherited the gene as well. She says that she will send each of her sisters a letter about her *BRCA1* results. Ms. Harris tells Mrs. Cohen that she has made a very important decision that will be helpful to her sisters.

Conclusion

The practice of nursing is now incorporating genetic and genomic information and technologies into all areas of practice, including the understanding and consideration of ethical issues. As such, nurses need to be able to identify the ethical, legal, and social issues related to genomic information and technologies. Nurses and other healthcare providers need to understand the principles of ethics and law, including human rights and human dignity, so that they will be able to handle complex healthcare issues. They need to be knowledgeable about genetic and genomic science and their influence on health care, including information about ethical issues such as informed consent, confidentiality and privacy of an individual's genetic information, and discrimination based on personal genetic information to ensure that patients and families are being provided appropriate health care. Nurses should maintain and update their genetic and genomic knowledge and competency in genomics, including the rapidly evolving ethical, legal, and social issues related to genomic health care (Badzek et al., 2013). To achieve this goal, nurses should become familiar with reliable resources that can help them integrate genetics and genomics and the relevant ethical issues into their practice (Lea, 2008). Figure 7-1 provides a list-

---

Figure 7-1. Genetic and Genomic Resources for Nurses

- American Nurses Association NursingWorld, Personalized Medicine: http://nursing world.org/MainMenuCategories/EthicsStandards/Genetics-1
- Centers for Disease Control and Prevention, Genomics and Health Resources (A–Z): www.cdc.gov/genomics/public/index.htm
- Genetics Home Reference, Your Guide to Understanding Genetic Conditions: http://ghr.nlm.nih.gov
- Genetics/Genomics Competency Center: www.g-2-c-2.org
- International Society of Nurses in Genetics: www.isong.org
- My Family Health Portrait: https://familyhistory.hhs.gov/FHH/html/index.html
- National Human Genome Research Institute
  - Genetic and Rare Diseases Information Center: www.genome.gov/10000409
  - Issues in Genetics: www.genome.gov/10000006
  - Issues in Genetics and Health: www.genome.gov/10001740
- Telling Stories: Understanding Real Life Genetics: www.tellingstories.nhs.uk

---

ing of important genomic resources for nurses that contain current genetic and genomic information relevant to health care.

References

American Academy of Pediatrics. (2013). Ethical and policy issues in genetic testing and screening of children [Policy statement]. *Pediatrics, 131,* 620–622. doi:10.1542/peds.2012-3680

American Academy of Pediatrics Committee on Bioethics. (2001). Ethical issues with genetic testing in children. *Pediatrics, 107,* 1451–1455. doi:10.1542/peds.107.6.1451

American Nurses Association. (2015). *Code of ethics for nurses with interpretive statements.* Retrieved from http://www.nursingworld.org/DocumentVault/Ethics_1/Code-of-Ethics-for-Nurses.html

Athena Diagnostics. (2013). Genetic testing policy. Retrieved from http://www.athenadiagnostics.com/content/ordering/genetic_testing

Badzek, L., Henaghan, M., Turner, M., & Monsen, R. (2013). Ethical, legal, and social issues in the translation of genomics into healthcare. *Journal of Nursing Scholarship, 45,* 15–24. doi:10.1111/jnu.12000

Beery, T.A., & Workman, M.L. (2012). *Genetics and genomics in nursing and health care.* Philadelphia, PA: F.A. Davis.

Consensus Panel on Genetic/Genomic Nursing Competencies. (2009). *Essentials of genetic and genomic nursing: Competencies, curricula guidelines, and outcome indicators* (2nd ed.). Silver Spring, MD: American Nurses Association.

Gallo, A.M., Angst, D.B., & Knafl, K.A. (2009). Disclosure of genetic information within families. *American Journal of Nursing, 109*(4), 65–69. doi:10.1097/01.NAJ.0000348607.31983.6e

Genetics Home Reference. (2014). What is a chromosome? Retrieved from http://ghr.nlm.nih.gov/handbook/basics/chromosome

Hudson, K., Javitt, G., Burke, W., Byers, P., & American Society of Human Genetics Social Issues Committee. (2007). ASHG statement on direct-to-consumer genetic testing in the United States. *American Journal of Human Genetics, 81,* 635–637. doi:10.1086/521634

International Council of Nurses. (2012). *The ICN code of ethics for nurses.* Retrieved from http://www.icn.ch/images/stories/documents/about/icncode_english.pdf

International Society of Nurses in Genetics. (2009). Direct-to-consumer marketing of genetic tests [Position statement]. Retrieved from http://www.isong.org/pdfs2013/PS_Marketing_Genetic_Tests.pdf

International Society of Nurses in Genetics. (2010). Privacy and confidentiality of genetic information: The role of the nurse [Position statement]. Retrieved from http://www.isong.org/pdfs2013/PS_Privacy_Confidentiality.pdf

Kaiser, J. (2012, October 11). President's ethics panel urges new protections for whole genome data. Retrieved from http://news.sciencemag.org/policy/2012/10/presidents-ethics-panel-urges-new-protections-whole-genome-data

Lea, D.H. (2008). Genetic and genomic healthcare: Ethical issues of importance to nurses. *Online Journal of Issues in Nursing, 13*, Manuscript 4. Retrieved from http://www.nursingworld.org/MainMenuCategories/ANAMarketplace/ANAPeriodicals/OJIN/TableofContents/vol132008/No1Jan08/GeneticandGenomicHealthcare.html

National Human Genome Research Institute. (2012a). Elements of informed consent described in federal regulations. Retrieved from http://www.genome.gov/27526659

National Human Genome Research Institute. (2012b). GAO concludes that DTC genetic tests mislead consumers. Retrieved from https://www.genome.gov/19518344

National Human Genome Research Institute. (2012c). An overview of the Human Genome Project. Retrieved from http://www.genome.gov/12011238

National Human Genome Research Institute. (2012d). Protecting human research subjects. Retrieved from http://www.genome.gov/10001752

National Human Genome Research Institute. (2014a). Frequently asked questions about genetic testing. Retrieved from http://www.genome.gov/19516567

National Human Genome Research Institute. (2014b). Genetic discrimination. Retrieved from http://www.genome.gov/Glossary/index.cfm?id=80

National Human Genome Research Institute. (2014c). Genetic Information Nondiscrimination Act of 2008. Retrieved from http://www.genome.gov/10002328

National Human Genome Research Institute. (2014d). Talking glossary of genetic terms: Genomics. Retrieved from http://www.genome.gov/Glossary/index.cfm?id=532

National Human Genome Research Institute. (2014e). Talking glossary of genetic terms: Personalized medicine. Retrieved from http://www.genome.gov/Glossary/index.cfm?id=150

National Human Genome Research Institute. (2014f). Talking glossary of genetic terms: Phenotype. Retrieved from http://www.genome.gov/Glossary/index.cfm?id=152

Seaman, A.M. (2013). Experts issue guidelines for gene tests in kids. Retrieved from http://www.reuters.com/article/2013/02/21/us-gene-tests-idUSBRE91K17620130221

U.S. Department of Health and Human Services. (n.d.). Understanding health information privacy. Retrieved from http://www.hhs.gov/ocr/privacy/hipaa/understanding/index.html

U.S. Department of Health and Human Services. (2009, April 6). *GINA: The Genetic Information Nondiscrimination Act of 2008: Information for researchers and health care professionals.* Retrieved from http://www.genome.gov/Pages/PolicyEthics/GeneticDiscrimination/GINAInfoDoc.pdf

CHAPTER 8

The Impact of Ethical Conflict and Dilemmas on Nurses

Melissa Kurtz, MSN, MA, RN, and Cynda Hylton Rushton, PhD, RN, FAAN

Introduction

Ethics has always been an integral part of nursing (Jameton, 1984), but several factors increase the likelihood that today's nurses will face ethical concerns as they participate in patient care. Advances in medical technology, an increased emphasis on patient self-determination, a focus on cost containment, recent healthcare reform legislation, and differing values among the stakeholders involved in providing patient care all are factors that can contribute to the rise of ethical concerns (Ong, Yee, & Lee, 2012). Understanding the types of ethical quandaries that can arise, the impact of such quandaries on the healthcare team, patient, and family, and how to address such conflicts is imperative to nurses' practice.

Because of the nature of the illnesses that they help to treat, oncology nurses are particularly likely to encounter moral concerns. Common ethical quandaries that oncology nurses might encounter include the following.
- What constitutes informed consent or truth telling (Cohen & Erickson, 2006)?
- How should end-of-life decision making proceed (Rice, Rady, Hamrick, Verheijde, & Pendergast, 2008)?
- Who is an ethically appropriate surrogate for the patient (Cohen & Erickson, 2006)?
- How should the benefits and burdens of cancer treatments be weighed in light of the patient's individualized prognosis (Smith, Lo, & Sudore, 2013)?

In addition, oncology nurses are frequently involved in caring for patients enrolled in clinical trials. Although such trials may help lead to the development of new cancer treatments, they also can have adverse effects on patients. Nurses involved in the care of patients enrolled in clinical trials may feel conflicted about facilitating such treatments (Shepard, 2010).

This chapter will begin with a case study drawn from the oncology setting that illustrates how ethical concerns may arise. Following the case study, the nature of various ethical concerns will be defined, along with responses to such ethical concerns. Finally, various causes of moral concerns and ways to address them will be discussed.

Case Study

Amelia Hutton, an 82-year-old retired teacher, was diagnosed six months ago with metastatic endometrial adenocarcinoma, which has spread to her lungs and adrenals. To date, she has undergone surgery and extensive chemotherapy. Recent scans reveal generalized regression of tumor size. She has tolerated the chemotherapy so far but has developed progressive complications including declining mental status with memory loss, peripheral neuropathy, and impaired vision. At her last doctor's visit, the oncologist recommends discontinuation of chemotherapy. Mrs. Hutton agrees with the recommendation, stating that she is overwhelmed with the treatments and very concerned about the impact of the complications on her ability to remain independent. She voices concern that she does not know how long she might live but wants to enjoy the time she has left.

Mrs. Hutton is married to Philip, 88, who also has significant chronic health problems, including osteoarthritis, hypertension, diabetes, and mild dementia. Mr. Hutton relies heavily on his wife for management of their home, health care, and activities of daily living. Together they have two adult children who live in distant cities. Mrs. Hutton has designated her husband as her healthcare agent.

Two days ago, Mrs. Hutton developed high fever, shaking chills, and disorientation. Mr. Hutton became frightened and called 911. Mrs. Hutton was taken to the emergency department and admitted for presumed sepsis. Fluids, antibiotics, and aggressive treatments were initiated. During the first 24 hours, she developed progressive respiratory distress that required oxygen, positive-pressure breathing support, and steroids. Today, her condition has continued to deteriorate with hemodynamic instability and worsening respiratory distress.

The clinical team is concerned that an intensive care unit admission may be needed and is anxious to clarify Mrs. Hutton's resuscitation status. When the team members explore this with her, they find her to have fluctuating decision-making capacity; at times she says that she wants to live as long as she can, whereas other times she states that she has suffered enough and is ready to "meet her maker." The intern on the case is unsure how to proceed, but is told by the attending physician to involve Mrs. Hutton's husband as the team deliberates her resuscitation status. When the intern asks Mr. Hutton what he thinks his wife would want, he states, "I don't want her to die—she's everything to me."

Discussion

Mrs. Hutton's case highlights the declining healthcare condition of an elderly woman with cancer and depicts the deliberation of her resuscitation status by the healthcare team. Her case provides an example of an ethically complex treatment decision that frequently arises in the healthcare setting, as well as a realistic context under which this decision must often be made. Resuscitation status is clearly important to patients, as they are the ones for whom this procedure is provided and because resuscitation can lead to varied outcomes. Initiating resuscitation sometimes restores a patient's functioning. In other cases, resuscitation procedures result in the sustaining of the patient's life, but at a decreased level of functioning. Still in other cases, resuscitation procedures can be unsuccessful, and the result is patient death.

The ultimate decision about a patient's resuscitation status also impacts the healthcare team in that they are the individuals who collaborate with the patient or the patient's surrogate to decide whether to carry out resuscitation. The outcome of resuscitation depends on several prognostic factors, which the healthcare team can help the patient or surrogate understand. If the decision is made to resuscitate the patient, members of the healthcare team are the ones who will carry out the procedure. When a patient desires resuscitation but the healthcare team feels that it will likely not sustain life, the healthcare team may feel distress in carrying out the patient's wishes.

Before Mrs. Hutton became ill and was hospitalized, she had independent decision-making capacity and expressed her healthcare goal and preference—to forgo further cancer treatment and maximize quality of life—to one of the doctors on her primary healthcare team. Mrs. Hutton also prepared for a time when she no longer had independent decision-making capacity by naming her husband as her healthcare agent. When Mrs. Hutton became ill at home and could no longer verbalize her own healthcare wishes, her husband became the person to make decisions on her behalf. Although the role of healthcare agents is to make decisions based on the patient's own expressed wishes, sometimes healthcare agents are unsure how the patient would decide in a particular instance. It is unclear whether Mr. Hutton understood his wife's healthcare goals and preferences, yet even if he did, he may have become distressed when his wife became ill at home, which resulted in him calling 911.

Once at the hospital, Mrs. Hutton is so ill that her decision-making capacity is fluctuating, which means that her husband is called upon to be involved in the decision about her resuscitation status. Even if Mr. Hutton had known his wife's wishes about resuscitation at this point in time, he may have found it difficult to honor such wishes because of his strong social and emotional ties to the patient. Mr. Hutton's reliance on his wife for household management and activities of daily living may have been influencing factors in his decision making about resuscitation when approached by the healthcare team. The healthcare team, another group of individuals involved in the resuscitation decision, may be unaware of Mrs. Hutton's prior conversations with her family and outpatient physicians, so it may be unclear to them how to share the decision-making burden of resuscitation status with Mr. Hutton as his wife's condition worsens. As a result, the team may be experiencing a number of ethical conflicts or dilemmas. The type of ethical dilemmas and conflicts that can arise in healthcare treatment decisions such as resuscitation will be discussed in the sections that follow, with application made to Mrs. Hutton's case.

Categories of Moral Concerns

In an early publication discussing nursing practice, Jameton (1984) offered a helpful distinction between the following moral concepts: *moral uncertainty*, *moral dilemma*, and *moral distress*. A fourth term, *moral conflict*, is also an important moral concern. These terms will be defined and discussed in the context of Mrs. Hutton's case.

Moral Uncertainty

Moral uncertainty occurs when a healthcare provider is unsure whether an ethical dilemma is present or is unclear what principles apply to an ethical dilemma (Jameton, 1984). Any healthcare provider could experience moral uncertainty. It may arise more often in early-career health professionals or in those with limited healthcare ethics training. In the case of Mrs. Hutton, the healthcare team seems to be exhibiting a level of moral uncertainty. The team members may be unsure how to frame the ethical tensions they are experiencing. It may not be clear who ought to make the decision about Mrs. Hutton's treatment and what ethical principles apply. Finding the language to express the concerns is often a key element in determining whether an ethical concern exists and the nature of it.

Moral Dilemma

A *moral dilemma* occurs when two or more ethical values or principles conflict, making it difficult to choose among the various options (Jameton, 1984). In the case of a moral dilemma, all options could be morally supportable, but only one can be chosen. In choosing one solution, an individual may feel that he or she is losing something valuable. In the healthcare setting, moral dilemmas arise because of the sometimes-competing values held by the individuals or organizations involved in providing care. For instance, the nursing profession, as with other health professions, has been characterized as "inherently moral," with clear ethical goals including the protection of patients, provision of care that prevents complications, and maintenance of a healing environment (Zuzelo, 2007). The patients and families for whom nurses care also have values and preferences that guide healthcare decision making. The patient's and family's values can be shaped by family traditions, cultural and spiritual beliefs, the media, previous healthcare experiences, general or healthcare knowledge, and other factors. Finally, healthcare systems have explicit values that inform their operations. When differences in values among these or other stakeholders arise, the care provider (i.e., nurse) may struggle to preserve all interests or values.

In Mrs. Hutton's case, the team may be struggling to balance respect for Mrs. Hutton's dignity and choices with concerns about her decision-making capacity and that of her surrogate, Mr. Hutton. They may question how her prior preferences relate to the current decisions and how her husband's preferences ought to impact the choices about ventilation and resuscitation as her own decision-making capacity fluctuates or is extinguished. Similarly, team members may be struggling with the balance of benefits and burdens as they attempt to understand what is medically possible and desired by Mrs. Hutton in light of the choices of her surrogate. Imbedded in these questions are conceptual and value-laden assessments of quality of life, suffering, and comfort.

Moral Conflict

When two or more stakeholders have different opinions about how a moral dilemma should be resolved, a *moral conflict* can result. Moral conflicts can arise between any number of involved stakeholders, such as between members of the healthcare team and the patient and/or family, between family members and the patient, or between different members within an individual family. Conflicts usually involve disagreements about the overall goals of care for the patient or the benefits of treatment to the individual (Education in Palliative and End-of-Life Care [EPEC] Project, 1999).

Conflicts are more likely to occur in cases where a communication breakdown has occurred. Communication breakdowns include instances where healthcare team members have not clearly communicated medical facts—perhaps because they have used medical jargon—or have conveyed different, conflicting information to a patient or family. For instance, when patients or families are initially given an optimistic prognosis but subsequently are given a different, grimmer prognosis, they may respond by clashing with members of the healthcare team if asked to discontinue treatments that are viewed as life sustaining (EPEC Project, 1999).

Moral conflicts also may arise because of various personal factors. For instance, if a patient or family distrusts the medical team, they may respond by disagreeing with the team's recommendations about a treatment decision. Grief, guilt, or memories of past experiences also may cause patients or families to become entrenched in their own positions, which may be different from those of the healthcare team. On rare occasions, family members who are acting as surrogate decision makers conflict with the medical team because they are seeking secondary gain. For example, a surrogate who will lose financial income after a patient dies may opt for continued life-sustaining treatments rather than comfort care (EPEC Project, 1999).

In the case of Mrs. Hutton, moral conflicts that might arise include conflicts about the patient's overall goals of care, resuscitation status, and individual treatment decision making for other medical issues. Moral conflict is more likely to occur in Mrs. Hutton's case if one individual or a group of stakeholders believes that the best ethical course of action for Mrs. Hutton is continued life-prolonging treatment, whereas another stakeholder believes that comfort care is the best course of action. Ideally, moral conflicts such as these can be addressed and resolved using strategies outlined later in this chapter.

If the ethical concerns highlighted in Mrs. Hutton's case are not resolved or are exacerbated, moral distress can ensue. Consider, for example, that team members are unable to clarify their concerns regarding Mrs. Hutton's decision-making capacity and the balance of benefits and burdens of treatment, and Mr. Hutton requests that they do "everything," including continue mechanical ventilation, vasopressors, and resuscitation. After several weeks of aggressive treatment, the team believes that performing such acts is causing disproportionate suffering and dishonoring the dignity of Mrs. Hutton. Such concerns, if ongoing, might lead to moral distress.

Moral Distress

Moral distress is one response to moral conflicts or dilemmas. Nurses in the oncology setting report higher levels of moral distress than nurses in other acute care specialties (de Veer, Francke, Struijs, & Willems, 2013). Moral distress is "the pain or anguish affecting the mind, body, or relationships in response to a situation in which the person is aware of a moral problem, acknowledges moral responsibility, and makes a moral judgment about the correct action; yet, as a result of real or perceived constraints, participates in perceived moral wrongdoing" (Nathaniel, 2002). Any healthcare professional may experience moral distress, but Jameton first discussed the concept in the nursing literature in 1984. Moral distress differs from other types of distress and from moral dilemmas in that it involves the perception that one's core values are being violated while at the same time having a feeling of being constrained from taking the course of action that is perceived to be ethically appropriate (Epstein & Hamric, 2009). As a result, the clinician's integrity and authenticity are undermined (Beumer, 2008).

One situation that can contribute to nurses' moral distress is witnessing the devaluation of patient or family values and wishes (Huffman & Rittenmeyer, 2012). In the cancer setting, when the medical team's aim is to cure the patient and life-sustaining treatments are recommended, respecting the patient's or family's wishes for comfort care may be difficult for team members when the prognosis is grim or terminal (Shepard, 2010). Alternatively, as in the case of Mrs. Hutton, the patient's family may request continued life-sustaining treatment such as cardiopulmonary resuscitation (CPR), creating conflict with other stakeholders who support a comfort care–only approach. In one study, Ferrell (2006) reported that conflicts related to code status, continuing life support, and artificial nutrition and hydration most commonly caused moral distress for nurses. Furthermore, spiritual or religious factors frequently influenced decision making for patients with cancer (Ferrell, 2006).

Another situation that commonly results in moral distress is nurses' perception that their care—or lack of care—is contributing to patient suffering (Huffman & Rittenmeyer, 2012). This may involve nurses performing what they perceive to be unnecessary tests or procedures (Lazzarin, Biondi, & Di Mauro, 2012). It also may involve the nurse's perception that he or she is unable to effectively manage a patient's pain because of a physician's refusal to order analgesics or a family's refusal to have analgesics administered (Lazzarin et al., 2012; Varcoe, Pauly, Storch, Newton, & Makaroff, 2012). Oncology nurses frequently cite pain management as a concern and a common contributor to their moral distress (Lazzarin et al., 2012; Varcoe, Pauly, Storch, et al., 2012). If these issues about the scope of Mrs. Hutton's treatment are not resolved, the nurses caring for her will have to address them.

Nurses experiencing moral distress may respond in various ways. Occasionally, moral distress will cause nurses to become more vigilant and provide more care. This response usually stems from feelings of guilt (Burston & Tuckett, 2013). More often, nurses respond with negative psychological emotions, including frustration, anger, guilt, anxiety, and depression (Storch et al., 2009). Feelings of anticipatory dread, diminished self-confidence or self-doubt, and diminished sense of purpose are also characteristic responses to moral distress (Burston & Tuckett, 2013). Such responses may cause a nurse to withdraw from patients, which can negatively impact the quality of patient care and lead to increased pain, longer hospital stays, and inadequate or inappropriate care (Lang, 2008). The impact of moral distress is also felt among healthcare team members. Moral distress often erodes communication, compromising effective teamwork and sometimes resulting in system workarounds (Rushton, 2006).

Other Responses to Moral Conflicts and Dilemmas

Moral Outrage

Moral outrage can be a consequence of unregulated or unresolved moral distress or personal distress (Rushton, 2013). It may be described as anger provoked by a perceived violation of an ethical standard such as fairness, respect, or beneficence (Batson et al., 2007; Wilkinson, 1988). Moral outrage often presents as "energy-draining frustration, anger, disgust, and powerlessness" (Pike, 1991, p. 351) and is usually directed toward an individual or group, rarely toward oneself (Goodenough, 1997). Situations that may eventually lead to moral outrage include experiencing threats to one's personal or professional role, identity, self-worth, or integrity; encountering beliefs or practices that are different than one's own; or facing challenges to the beliefs, values, or preferences that define oneself (Rushton, 2013). When ungrounded and unexamined, moral outrage can exacerbate conflicts or differences that arise among stakeholders. When informed by wisdom, empathy, and compassion, moral outrage may be called "principled" and can become a tool for reestablishing a moral standard or value that the nurse perceives has been violated (Rushton, 2013).

Moral outrage can result in either action or inaction by the nurse (Rushton, 2013). For instance, in the oncology context, a nurse may perceive that her professional identity is jeopardized when asked to participate in treatment provision that fails to relieve the patient's suffering or that threatens to undermine the patient's values or preferences. A CPR attempt is one example that might meet either or both of these criteria. The nurse who participates in a resuscitation attempt under these conditions may perceive that her ethical obligations to do no harm, relieve suffering, and provide care that is in the patient's best interests are being violated. Such a perception may lead to the nurse experiencing moral outrage. If this moral outrage remains unexamined, it could lead to "depletion of vital energy, physical and emotional symptoms, unprofessional behaviors, and erosion of teamwork and patient centeredness" (Rushton, 2013, p. 84). Alternatively, the nurse may fail to advocate for what she feels is a violation of either her own professional values or the patient's values and become silent and apathetic (Rushton, 2013). If informed by empathy, wisdom, and compassion, the nurse's moral outrage could lead to a different approach, one where the nurse acts in a way to help resolve the moral dilemma or conflict that has arisen.

Burnout

Ongoing moral conflicts and moral dilemmas also can lead to burnout. Burnout is "a state of physical, emotional and mental exhaustion caused by long-term involvement in emotionally demanding situations" (Malakh-Pines & Aronson, 1998, p. 9). Burnout usually occurs gradually and is characterized by a range of symptoms, from mild, short-term disturbances (Rushton, Kaszniak, & Halifax, 2013) to high levels of emotional exhaustion, feelings of personal ineffectiveness or accomplishment, and high levels of depersonalization, cynicism, or detachment. Nurses who experience burnout may report decreased job satisfaction, choose to resign from a position, or leave the nursing profession altogether (Varcoe, Pauly, Webster, & Storch, 2012).

Although nurses in the oncology setting report experiences of burnout, burnout may be less dependent on setting than nursing demographics and the level of organizational support available. Nurses who had strong peer relationships and an environment in which to share their patient care experiences and resulting emotions reported that these positive coping strategies helped to prevent emotional exhaustion and feelings of depersonalization. Spirituality was also a positive coping strategy for some nurses and helped to prevent burnout (Davis, Lind, & Sorensen, 2013).

Contributing Factors to Moral Concerns

The previously described types of moral concerns arise because of a complex interplay of personal and organizational factors (Epstein & Hamric, 2009). In the following sections, various personal and organizational causes of moral concerns are discussed. They will be applied more generally to the issue of ethical conflict and specifically to the issue of moral distress, as much literature addresses this moral concern in depth.

Personal Causes
Worldview/Perception

A healthcare provider's worldview, or the ideas and beliefs through which one interprets and interacts with the world, will shape the way in which one understands and responds to moral concerns that arise through the course of providing patient care. An individual's worldview may be shaped by personal qualities or character traits (who the individual is and what his or her perceptions of events are), cultural background, life or personal experiences, or interpersonal relationships (Burston & Tuckett, 2013). An individual's worldview shapes his or her personal value system, which will be carried into the work setting where others may have different value systems. The literature notes specific factors related to worldview that can affect a nurse's level of moral distress. One study reported that nurses who were more influenced by their religious beliefs scored higher levels of moral distress than nurses whose personal value systems were influenced by factors such as family values, political views, life and work experiences, or professional codes of ethics (Davis, Schrader, & Belcheir, 2012).

Past Professional Experience

Studies are conflicted in terms of how one's years of nursing practice influence levels of moral distress. Some studies have reported that factors such as years of experience have no impact (de Veer et al., 2013), whereas other studies have suggested otherwise. Elpern, Covert, and Kleinpell (2005) reported a positive correlation between years of professional nursing practice and moral distress. Similarly, Epstein and Hamric (2009) proposed the concepts of moral distress (initial, acute distress occurring in the moment) and moral residue (reactive distress that remains after the initial distress is experienced) and posited that moral residue continues to rise over time (the crescendo effect), meaning that nurses who have been practicing longer may experience more distress and burnout. The authors cited three responses to increasing moral residue: (a) numbing of moral sensitivity and withdrawal from ethically challenging situations, (b) conscientious objection, and (c) burnout and departure from the nursing profession (Epstein & Hamric, 2009).

Perhaps more influential than one's years of nursing experience is how an individual's perceived level of skill and confidence in the clinical setting affect moral distress. Nurses who identify themselves as being highly confident and skilled tend to have lower levels of moral distress (Burston & Tuckett, 2013), whereas nurses who lack assertiveness or have self-doubt may have higher levels of moral distress (Epstein & Hamric, 2009).

Perceived Powerlessness

Healthcare environments can engender or sustain hierarchical relationships among the various healthcare professions, which can contribute to moral concerns. Although nurses have close proximity to patients at the bedside, they often feel they have less influence than other healthcare providers, especially physicians, in directing patient care. When faced with a situation in which powerlessness is felt, a nurse may respond by saying, "My opinion means nothing" (Varcoe, Pauly, Storch, et al., 2012). Demeaning messages or comments may reinforce feelings of powerlessness, as will angry outbursts aimed at the nurse (Varcoe, Pauly, Storch, et al., 2012). The socialization of nurses to follow orders may add to a sense of perceived powerlessness (Epstein & Hamric, 2009).

Some nurses who reported feeling a lack of recognition also acknowledged that the authority of the physician was not questioned (Huffman & Rittenmeyer, 2012). When nurses felt an increased responsibility for, or contribution to, the care of patients or families but lacked the authority to influence patient care decisions, moral distress increased. The perceived hierarchy between physicians and nurses kept the nurses from acting on their own moral position, which often differed from that of the physicians (Huffman & Rittenmeyer, 2012).

Organizational Causes
Scarce Resources

Moral concerns sometimes arise because of limited available resources. Nurses who encounter a shortage in material supplies or other resources needed to carry out patient care may feel unable to meet professional obligations to patients. When faced with scarce resources, nurses also may feel that their core values are unable to be upheld. Examples of limited resources that might contribute to moral dilemmas or moral distress include insufficient bed spaces, inadequate supplies, and inadequate care environments, such as lack of bereavement or palliative care space (Burston & Tuckett, 2013).

Insufficient staff and inadequately trained staff are other examples of scarce resources (Lazzarin et al., 2012). Unsafe staffing levels are responsible for triggering some of the highest levels of moral distress among nurses. Staff shortages prevent nurses from providing required care and contribute to a frenzied work pace, exhaustion, and feelings of demoralization (Burston & Tuckett, 2013). Staff shortages also can prevent nurses from attending in-services and educational sessions aimed at improving patient care during the workday (Rodney et al., 2002).

Lack of Collegial and Team Relationships

Nursing input in patients' plans of care is valuable because nurses spend long periods of time at the bedside and are keenly aware of moral concerns that arise. Despite this fact, nurses report frequent exclusion from discussions about patients' treatment goals with the healthcare team and may fail to have information that is key to resolving ethical conflicts or dilemmas (Hamric & Blackhall, 2007). Such lack of collaboration among team members can cause omissions in care, poor use of valuable resources, and conflicting advice or education to patients and family members (Burston & Tuckett, 2013). Moreover, nurses who lack the opportunity to be involved in ethical deliberations and care planning generally have higher levels of moral distress because they must implement care plans on which they had little input and may not support (McDaniel, 1998).

Lack of Leadership and Peer Support

The amount of practice support that a nurse receives is another factor that impacts moral distress. Moral distress is influenced by the availability of supportive leadership or supervision (de Veer et al., 2013). Absence of leadership and management in the clinical setting contributes to nurses' experiences of moral distress (Storch et al., 2009).

Studies of nurses in certain clinical settings have shown that peer support is also a crucial element in sustaining nursing practice. Bakker, LeBlanc, and Schaufeli (2005) concluded that intensive care unit nurses who reported the highest prevalence of burnout among their colleagues were most likely to experience high levels of burnout themselves. These findings suggest that at least in the critical care setting (but likely other settings as well), nurses' support or lack of support of one another has important consequences (Epp, 2012).

Values and Policies Governing the Healthcare Institution

A nurse's perception of the way an organization views and addresses ethical issues will impact the level of distress experienced (de Veer et al., 2013). Some studies report that institutional environments that overemphasize efficiency, effectiveness, and cost saving constrain nurses' ethical practice and contribute to moral distress (Pauly, Varcoe, Storch, & Newton, 2009). Nurses report more distress when the ultimate goal of the institution seems to be getting a procedure done rather than attending to patient well-being, interdisciplinary cohesion, and nurse satisfaction (Rodney et al., 2002). In addition, when a hospital's policies and practices conflict with evolving evidence-based practice, nurses may have increased distress. Nurses may feel that such policies constrain them from taking the action perceived to be most ethically appropriate (Burston & Tuckett, 2013).

Fear of Litigation

In the course of caring for patients, healthcare providers may encounter real or perceived threats of litigation. Fears of being sued can lead clinicians to provide treatment that appears "thorough" from a legal point of view but may not generate new clinical information that will benefit the patient (Rentmeester, 2008). As a result, patients may end up enduring unnecessary tests or procedures. Nurses who are responsible for performing or facilitating these tests or procedures but feel they are unnecessary may respond with increased levels of moral distress (Shepard, 2010).

Building Capacity to Address Moral Concerns

Individual

Ideally, moral conflict and dilemmas will be addressed and resolved and result in the growth of a nurse's ethical practice.

Self-Reflection and Self-Care

Nurses, who spend so much of their time engaged in patient care, which can give rise to moral distress, need time and training in how to self-reflect on the effects of their professional work. Critical self-reflection may serve many functions. One benefit of critical self-reflection is that it may allow nurses to identify or develop the skills needed to maintain their work in health care (Burston & Tuckett, 2013). Rushton (2009) discussed one tool that can aid a nurse's critical self-reflection practice: the art of pause. The art of pause involves taking a moment to stop, listen, and reflect more deeply on a situation. Pausing creates an opportunity to understand the meaning behind the spoken words, allows time to formulate questions, which can bring clarity, and gives space for seeing alternative viewpoints (Rushton, 2009). In addition to the art of pause, nurses may find journaling a helpful way to self-reflect (Murray, 2005).

Personal strategies for reducing moral distress also include healthy lifestyle choices, such as eating regular, well-balanced meals, getting enough rest, limiting caffeine and alcohol intake, and taking small, frequent breaks or vacations when able. More formal individualized practices for reducing moral distress might include courses in communication or stress management (Murray, 2005).

Conscientious Objection

When a nurse's moral integrity is violated such that the nurse experiences moral distress and subsequent moral outrage, and efforts to resolve the moral distress remain unsuccessful, one possible response of the nurse, as proposed in the literature, is conscientious objection. Conscientious objection is the refusal of a provider (i.e., nurse) to participate in certain types of care based on the fact that these care activities violate the provider's personal ethical beliefs (Davis et al.,

2012). The nurse's right to conscientiously object is supported legally in most states and professionally in the American Nurses Association's (ANA's) *Code of Ethics for Nurses* (2015). The ANA statement provides guidance on the types of situations where conscientious objection is justified.

> When nurses are placed in situations of compromise that exceed moral limits or that violate moral standards in any nursing practice setting, they must express to the appropriate authority their conscientious objection to participation in these situations. When a particular decision or action is morally objectionable to the nurse, whether intrinsically so or because it may jeopardize a specific patient, family, community, or population, or when it may jeopardize nursing practice, the nurse is justified in refusing to participate on moral grounds. Conscience-based refusals to participate exclude personal preference, prejudice, bias, convenience, or arbitrariness. (ANA, 2015, p. 20)

Others noted that conscientious objection could be a valid response by the nurse when he or she feels that a particular treatment or patient care action is particularly harmful (Davis et al., 2012). Catlin et al. (2008) proposed conscientious objection as one possible response in neonatal intensive care unit nurses, especially in cases where a nurse is asked to continue to carry out life-prolonging measures instead of comfort care–only measures for infants who are at the end of life.

According to Rushton (2013), a hallmark of principled moral outrage is an uncompromising commitment to uphold the highest ethical values and principles, which may involve conscientiously objecting in a respectful manner in certain instances. The author noted that it is necessary to determine "personal and collective thresholds of accommodation of morally distressing situations" (Rushton, 2013, p. 85). The various responses to violations of conscience include finding a compromise that preserves integrity, raising awareness about a violation of an ethical standard, refusing to participate, and exiting from a situation or institution where efforts to address instances leading to moral outrage remain unresolved (Rushton, 2013).

Organizational
Professional Standards and Guidelines

Various nursing organizations have addressed the phenomenon of moral distress as a key moral concern affecting the nursing workforce. The American Association of Critical-Care Nurses (AACN) calls for nurses to recognize the experience of moral distress, be knowledgeable about professional and institutional resources, and commit to addressing moral distress. A tool called "The 4 A's to Rise Above Moral Distress" is available online at www.aacn.org/WD/Practice/Docs/4As_to_Rise_Above_Moral_Distress.pdf. This tool encourages nurses to (a) Ask, or become aware of moral distress, (b) Affirm, or validate the distress and commit to address it, (c) Assess the sources of the distress, and (d) Act to address the distress. AACN also calls for organizations to create support systems, develop processes for analyzing systems issues that enable moral distress, and provide education and tools to manage moral distress (AACN, 2008).

Engagement in Political Advocacy and Action

For some nurses, engagement in political advocacy or action groups is a helpful way to address moral distress. Specifically, political action is a way of addressing some of the structural and organizational issues that contribute to moral distress (Varcoe, Pauly, Storch, et al., 2012). Nurses at every level of organizational practice can be involved in shaping health policy so that it is more supportive of nurses' ethical practice (Rodney et al., 2002). An example of a political advocacy activity in which nurses can engage is lobbying efforts aimed at resource funding, such as staffing or workforce issues (Burston & Tuckett, 2013).

Clear Organizational Policies

Developing institutional policies that address issues that have ethical implications provides a framework for all clinicians, including nurses, and may diminish ambiguity when providing patient care, subsequently diminishing moral distress. Clinical brain death is one example where having an institutional policy can prove to be helpful in minimizing moral distress. Brain death is a relatively infrequent but devastating diagnosis made through confirmatory testing and procedures, but the criteria for making such a determination can vary, and family members from certain religious backgrounds may disagree with the criteria set forth by the healthcare team. Formulating an institutional policy clarifies the clinical procedures for diagnosing brain death and offers guidelines on how to proceed if family members disagree with the diagnosis.

Forgoing life-sustaining treatment, a common decision that arises in the oncology setting, is another situation for which having an institutional policy can be beneficial. State laws vary in terms of how decision making for the removal of life-sustaining treatment should proceed. Clarifying in a policy who can make such decisions and how such decisions should go forward helps the medical team navigate end-of-life care concerns. Such policies also may help to ease the moral distress that nurses and clinicians experience during end-of-life decision making.

Chaplaincy and Hospital Support Services

For some nurses, addressing moral distress might be aided by use of chaplaincy or other support services (Burston & Tuckett, 2013). Even if large, group-facilitated discussions aimed at addressing moral distress are part of a unit's practice, individuals may not feel comfortable exploring their own distress in such a setting. Making available a counselor, grief team, psychologist, or religious services people to nursing staff is one way to provide individualized support.

Developing Skills and Capacities

Nurses need the ability to navigate ethical decisions when challenging situations arise, which means having tools to engage in treatment decision-making discussions where differing opinions among stakeholders may exist (Burston & Tuckett, 2013). Nurses often find it difficult to participate in discussions with the healthcare team because of underlying professional hierarchies, particularly among physicians and nurses (MacKintosh & Sandall, 2010). One way to address professional hierarchies is by finding ways to better communicate with other disciplines that are distinct but have shared patient interests.

Standardized communication protocols such as SBAR (Situation, Background, Assessment, Recommendation) are one way of facilitating communication between nurses and physicians. Communication protocols were originally crafted for use in emergency situations where articulation of concerns must happen quickly and, more often than not, via telecommunication (MacKintosh & Sandall, 2010). Some research suggests that standardized communication tools not only facilitate communication between nurses and physicians in emergency situations but also positively impact the healthcare environment by allowing rapid decision making by nurses, providing social capital and legitimacy for less-tenured nurses, and reinforcing a move toward standardization in the nursing profession (Vardaman et al., 2012). By providing a way of communicating that empowers nurses in their clinical role, standardized communication tools may help to diminish levels of moral distress.

Nurses also will benefit from developing skills in moral reasoning and decision making. These skills can be achieved through ethics education forums or classes offered by either the institution or outside organizations. Developing skills in conflict resolution or mediation can be especially helpful. Moral conflicts arise because of disagreements about the appropriate plan of care for a patient. The goal of mediation is to address stakeholders' discomforts about care planning and find consensus among those who disagree (Dubler, 2011).

Team Collaboration

Recommendations for addressing moral distress include providing opportunities for healthcare professionals to engage in reflective dialogue and share stories with colleagues (Mitton, Peacock, Storch, Smith, & Cornelissen, 2010). The format for these dialogues might take the shape of unit debriefings, where all involved team members gather to discuss the impact of a certain case or event (Shepard, 2010). The process of talking about morally distressing cases or situations can, in and of itself, be therapeutic (Mitton et al., 2010). Although the environment for such interprofessional discussions is not a place where all aspects of moral distress can be addressed, the forum is a place where the plan for addressing organizational factors that contribute to moral distress can begin to take shape. Following the group conversation, leadership can more thoroughly explore why the distress happened, considering interpersonal, interdisciplinary, unit, and institutional factors (Rushton, 2006). The goal of this space is to provide an opportunity for various individuals' questions and perceptions to be voiced and heard (Mitton et al., 2010).

Strengthening physician–nurse collaboration is also important and takes concerted effort (Hamric & Blackhall, 2007). Some techniques that might facilitate better collaboration include communication and other seminars aimed at fostering teamwork and interdisciplinary forums in a safe setting where respectful discussion can happen.

After-hours social events for staff are another way to build collaboration and facilitate an environment of sharing (Gutierrez, 2005). Supportive peer relationships can reduce elements such as burnout that contribute to moral distress (Bakker et al., 2005). Peers also can help nurses address the ethical quandaries that arise through the course of providing patient care (Rodney et al., 2002). The organization of a buddy system, where two nurses regularly provide support and encouragement to one another, or nursing staff awards given based on nominations from peers or colleagues, are other ways to promote nursing collaboration (McClendon & Buckner, 2007). Finally, creating an environment where nurses at all levels of the organization can discuss ethical concerns offers a sense of connection for nurses (Storch et al., 2009).

Supportive Leadership

Support from nursing leadership or management can impact the clinical environment in positive ways, minimizing factors that can lead to moral distress. Nurses in formal leadership roles are key in helping to create a supportive environment where dialogue about ethical situations can occur (Storch et al., 2009). The chief nursing officer (or other nursing administrator) seems particularly influential in helping nurses feel understood and heard and in conveying that ethical issues are important within the institution (Storch et al., 2009).

Nurse leaders are perceived as supportive when they help negotiate the interactions between nursing and other disciplines on the unit and promptly respond to requests (Varcoe, Pauly, Storch, et al., 2012). An overall leadership style that is more relational rather than focused on tasks leads to higher nurse satisfaction; ultimately, the nurse leader's style can help to buffer the intensity of moral distress that a nurse experiences (de Veer et al., 2013).

Nursing leadership can provide support in at least two important ways. First, managers can regularly make themselves available to nurses at the bedside. Coles (2010) noted that nurses often feel a sense of support and understanding when management is visibly present on the unit and helps with patient care planning or with brainstorming patient care interventions. Managers also can accomplish better presence on the unit through daily rounds with the charge nurse. By making themselves available for patient care issues and getting to know the nursing staff on the unit, nurse managers can recognize and address signs of moral distress before negative consequences result (Coles, 2010). One intervention that nurse leaders can take is to identify mentors for nurses working on their units. Having such support is key in reducing moral distress (Burston & Tuckett, 2013).

Another intervention is to rotate patient assignments to lessen the burden of moral distress of nurses caring for complex patients (Shepard, 2010). Some nurse leaders in the oncology setting organize cancer survivor days, which allow nurses to visit with former patients and see the outcome of their care (Shepard, 2010). Witnessing the progress of former patients can provide encouragement and a sense of professional fulfillment for nurses.

Second, nurse managers can facilitate collegial relationships among various disciplines (Epp, 2012). For instance, nurse managers can offer a nursing perspective in conversations with physicians, thereby bringing attention to nursing-specific issues that need to be addressed (Manojlovich & Laschinger, 2008). Studies confirm that nursing leadership can influence the extent to which nurses and physicians on a unit collaborate, as well as unit staffing levels, both of which subsequently affect levels of emotional exhaustion, feelings of depersonalization, the sense of personal accomplishment experienced by nursing staff, and the likelihood that nurses will remain in their current position (Leiter & Laschinger, 2006). Interventions that nurse managers might take to facilitate nurse–physician collaboration include being available to call a physician to discuss a patient care concern or to examine a patient (Varcoe, Pauly, Storch, et al., 2012).

Access to Ethics Education or Resources

Ethics education is a way of addressing and strengthening both individual and organizational responses to moral concerns (Pauly et al., 2009). At the individual level, ethics education can help practitioners to understand and develop strategies for coping with moral concerns, including moral distress (Burston & Tuckett, 2013). Ethics education seems to positively influence an individual practitioner's moral confidence and moral action (Burston & Tuckett, 2013).

Ethics education that includes techniques for fostering interprofessional collaboration and strengthening aspects of the clinical environment is also important in terms of addressing organizational or systems issues linked to moral distress (Burston & Tuckett, 2013). As discussed previously, interprofessional educational forums where various disciplines gather together to understand the different decision-making approaches to patient care in light of patient goals can help to facilitate collaboration (Burston & Tuckett, 2013). Other techniques for facilitating interprofessional education include role plays, where interdisciplinary professionals enact various clinical scenarios; ethics rounds, where case-specific or other moral concepts are taught to all team members; and storytelling or guided reflection, where team members have space to describe or discuss experiences that triggered moral concerns or distress (Burston & Tuckett, 2013).

Institutional ethics committees also may be a resource for nurses. The primary functions of ethics committees are education, case consultation, and policy development (Mercurio, 2011). Although not all nurses can be members of ethics committees or take part in meetings, this venue may be a place for nurses to have representation and to voice their ethical decision-making concerns and process. Similarly, institutional ethics consultation services can help nurses and other team members understand the ethical issues involved in a given case as well as facilitate discussion and offer recommendations (Mercurio, 2011).

Conclusion

Nurses in the oncology setting will continue to encounter the ethical conflicts and dilemmas identified in this chapter. In fact, as technology advances and healthcare treatments change, other ethical dilemmas may arise. The goal of the material presented here is to offer oncology nurses a foundational understanding of ethical conflicts and dilemmas as presently understood, as well as various means for addressing such dilemmas. In doing so, the hope is that oncology nurses will be better able to sustain their ethical practice at the bedside and their crucial role within the context of the healthcare team.

References

American Association of Critical-Care Nurses. (2008, August). Moral distress [Position statement]. Retrieved from http://www.aacn.org/WD/practice/Docs/moral_distress.pdf

American Nurses Association. (2015). Code of ethics for nurses with interpretive statements. Retrieved from http://www.nursingworld.org/MainMenuCategories/EthicsStandards/CodeofEthicsforNurses/Code-of-Ethics.html

Bakker, A.B., Le Blanc, P.M., & Schaufeli, W.B. (2005). Burnout contagion among intensive care nurses. Journal of Advanced Nursing, 51, 276–287. doi:10.1111/j.1365-2648.2005.03494.x

Batson, C.D., Kennedy, C.L., Nord, L., Stocks, E.L., Fleming, D.A., Marzette, C.M., ... Zerger, T. (2007). Anger at unfairness: Is it moral outrage? European Journal of Social Psychology, 37, 1272–1285. doi:10.1002/ejsp.434

Beumer, C.M. (2008). Innovative solutions: The effect of a workshop on reducing the experience of moral distress in an intensive care unit setting. Dimensions of Critical Care Nursing, 27, 263–267. doi:10.1097/01.DCC.0000338871.77658.03

Burston, A.S., & Tuckett, A.G. (2013). Moral distress in nursing: Contributing factors, outcomes and interventions. Nursing Ethics, 20, 312–324. doi:10.1177/0969733012462049

Catlin, A., Volat, D., Hadley, M.A., Bassir, R., Armigo, C., Valle, E., ... Anderson, K. (2008). Conscientious objection: A potential neonatal nursing response to care orders that cause suffering at the end of life? Study of a concept. Neonatal Network, 27, 101–108. doi:10.1891/0730-0832.27.2.101

Cohen, J.S., & Erickson, J.M. (2006). Ethical dilemmas and moral distress in oncology nursing practice. Clinical Journal of Oncology Nursing, 10, 775–780. doi:10.1188/06.CJON.775-780

Coles, D. (2010). "Because we can . . .": Leadership responsibility and the moral distress dilemma. Nursing Management, 41(3), 26–30. doi:10.1097/01.NUMA.0000369495.69358.dc

Davis, S., Lind, B.K., & Sorensen, C. (2013). A comparison of burnout among oncology nurses working in adult and pediatric inpatient and outpatient settings [Online exclusive]. Oncology Nursing Forum, 40, E303–E311. doi:10.1188/13.ONF.E303-E311

Davis, S., Schrader, V., & Belcheir, M.J. (2012). Influencers of ethical beliefs and the impact on moral distress and conscientious objection. Nursing Ethics, 19, 738–749. doi:10.1177/0969733011423409

de Veer, A.J., Francke, A.L., Struijs, A., & Willems, D.L. (2013). Determinants of moral distress in daily nursing practice: A cross sectional correlational questionnaire survey. International Journal of Nursing Studies, 50, 100–108. doi:10.1016/j.ijnurstu.2012.08.017

Dubler, N.N. (2011). A principled resolution: The fulcrum for bioethics resolution. *Law and Contemporary Problems, 74,* 177–200.

Education in Palliative and End-of-Life Care Project. (1999). *Education for Physicians on End-of-Life Care (EPEC) participant's handbook. Module 9: Medical futility.* Retrieved from http://endlink.lurie.northwestern.edu/medical_futility/module9.pdf

Elpern, E.H., Covert, B., & Kleinpell, R. (2005). Moral distress of staff nurses in a medical intensive care unit. *American Journal of Critical Care, 14,* 523–530.

Epp, K. (2012). Burnout in critical care nurses: A literature review. *Dynamics, 23*(4), 25–31.

Epstein, E.G., & Hamric, A.B. (2009). Moral distress, moral residue, and the crescendo effect. *Journal of Clinical Ethics, 20,* 330–352.

Ferrell, B.R. (2006). Understanding the moral distress of nurses witnessing medically futile care. *Oncology Nursing Forum, 33,* 922–930. doi:10.1188/06.ONF.922-930

Goodenough, W.H. (1997). Moral outrage: Territoriality in human guise. *Zygon, 32,* 5–27. doi:10.1111/0591-2385.671997067

Gutierrez, K.M. (2005). Critical care nurses' perceptions of and responses to moral distress. *Dimensions of Critical Care Nursing, 24,* 229–241. doi:10.1097/00003465-200509000-00011

Hamric, A.B., & Blackhall, L.J. (2007). Nurse-physician perspectives on the care of dying patients in intensive care units: Collaboration, moral distress, and ethical climate. *Critical Care Medicine, 35,* 422–429. doi:10.1097/01.CCM.0000254722.50608.2D

Huffman, D.M., & Rittenmeyer, L. (2012). How professional nurses working in hospital environments experience moral distress: A systematic review. *Critical Care Nursing Clinics of North America, 24,* 91–100. doi:10.1016/j.ccell.2012.01.004

Jameton, A. (1984). *Nursing practice: The ethical issues.* Englewood Cliffs, NJ: Prentice Hall.

Lang, K.R. (2008). The professional ills of moral distress and nurse retention: Is ethics education an antidote? *American Journal of Bioethics, 8*(4), 19–21. doi:10.1080/15265160802147181

Lazzarin, M., Biondi, A., & Di Mauro, S. (2012). Moral distress in nurses in oncology and haematology units. *Nursing Ethics, 19,* 183–195. doi:10.1177/0969733011416840

Leiter, M.P., & Laschinger, H.K.S. (2006). Relationships of work and practice environment to professional burnout: Testing a causal model. *Nursing Research, 55,* 137–146. doi:10.1097/00006199-200603000-00009

MacKintosh, N., & Sandall, J. (2010). Overcoming gendered and professional hierarchies in order to facilitate escalation of care in emergency situations: The role of standardised communication protocols. *Social Science and Medicine, 71,* 1683–1686. doi:10.1016/j.socscimed.2010.07.037

Malakh-Pines, A., & Aronson, E. (1988). *Career burnout: Causes and cures.* New York, NY: Free Press.

Manojlovich, M., & Laschinger, H.K.S. (2008). Application of the Nursing Worklife Model to the ICU setting. *Critical Care Nursing Clinics of North America, 20,* 481–487. doi:10.1016/j.ccell.2008.08.004

McClendon, H., & Buckner, E.B. (2007). Distressing situations in the intensive care unit: A descriptive study of nurses' responses. *Dimensions of Critical Care Nursing, 26,* 199–206.

McDaniel, C. (1998). Ethical environment: Reports of practicing nurses. *Nursing Clinics of North America, 32,* 363–372.

Mercurio, M.R. (2011). The role of a pediatric ethics committee in the newborn intensive care unit. *Journal of Perinatology, 31,* 1–9.

Mitton, C., Peacock, S., Storch, J., Smith, N., & Cornelissen, E. (2010). Moral distress among healthcare managers: Conditions, consequences and potential responses. *Healthcare Policy, 6*(2), 99–112. doi:10.12927/hcpol.2010.22036

Murray, R. (2005). *Managing your stress: A guide for nurses.* Retrieved from https://www2.rcn.org.uk/__data/assets/pdf_file/0008/78515/001484.pdf

Nathaniel, A. (2002). Moral distress among nurses. *American Nurses Association Ethics and Human Rights Issues Update, 2*(1).

Ong, W.Y., Yee, C.M., & Lee, A. (2012). Ethical dilemmas in the care of cancer patients near the end of life. *Singapore Medical Journal, 53,* 11–16.

Pauly, B., Varcoe, C., Storch, J., & Newton, L. (2009). Registered nurses' perceptions of moral distress and ethical climate. *Nursing Ethics, 16*, 561–573. doi:10.1177/0969733009106649

Pike, A.W. (1991). Moral outrage and moral discourse in nurse-physician collaboration. *Journal of Professional Nursing, 7*, 351–362. doi:10.1016/8755-7223(91)90012-A

Rentmeester, C.A. (2008). Moral damage to health care professionals and trainees: Legalism and other consequences for patients and colleagues. *Journal of Medicine and Philosophy, 33*, 27–43. doi:10.1093/jmp/jhm006

Rice, E.M., Rady, M.Y., Hamrick, A., Verheijde, J.L., & Pendergast, D.K. (2008). Determinants of moral distress in medical and surgical nurses at an adult acute tertiary care hospital. *Journal of Nursing Management, 16*, 360–373. doi:10.1111/j.1365-2834.2007.00798.x

Rodney, P., Varcoe, C., Storch, J.L., McPherson, G., Mahoney, K., Brown, H., … Starzomski, R. (2002). Navigating towards a moral horizon: A multisite qualitative study of ethical practice in nursing. *Canadian Journal of Nursing Research, 34*, 75–102.

Rushton, C.H. (2006). Defining and addressing moral distress: Tools for critical care nursing leaders. *AACN Advanced Critical Care, 17*, 161–168. doi:10.1097/00044067-200604000-00011

Rushton, C.H. (2009). Ethical discernment and action: The art of pause. *AACN Advanced Critical Care, 20*, 108–111. doi:10.1097/NCI.0b013e31819455dd

Rushton, C.H. (2013). Principled moral outrage: An antidote to moral distress? *AACN Advanced Critical Care, 24*, 82–89. doi:10.1097/NCI.0b013e31827b7746

Rushton, C.H., Kaszniak, A.W., & Halifax, J.S. (2013). A framework for understanding moral distress among palliative care clinicians. *Journal of Palliative Medicine, 16*, 1074–1079. doi:10.1089/jpm.2012.0490

Shepard, A. (2010). Moral distress: A consequence of caring. *Clinical Journal of Oncology Nursing, 14*, 25–27. doi:10.1188/10.CJON.25-27

Smith, A.K., Lo, B., & Sudore, R. (2013). When previously expressed wishes conflict with best interests. *JAMA Internal Medicine, 173*, 1241–1245.

Storch, J., Rodney, P., Varcoe, C., Pauly, B., Starzomski, R., Stevenson, L., … Newton, L. (2009). Leadership for Ethical Policy and Practice (LEPP): Participatory action project. *Nursing Leadership, 22*(3), 68–80. doi:10.12927/cjnl.2009.21155

Varcoe, C., Pauly, B., Storch, J., Newton, L., & Makaroff, K. (2012). Nurses' perceptions of and responses to morally distressing situations. *Nursing Ethics, 19*, 488–500. doi:10.1177/0969733011436025

Varcoe, C., Pauly, B., Webster, G., & Storch, J. (2012). Moral distress: Tensions as springboards for action. *HEC Forum, 24*, 51–62. doi:10.1007/s10730-012-9180-2

Vardaman, J.M., Cornell, P., Gondo, M.B., Amis, J.M., Townsend-Gervis, M., & Thetford, C. (2012). Beyond communication: The role of standardized protocols in a changing health care environment. *Health Care Management Review, 37*, 88–97. doi:10.1097/HMR.0b013e31821fa503

Wilkinson, J.M. (1988). Moral distress in nursing practice: Experience and effect. *Nursing Forum, 23*, 16–29. doi:10.1111/j.1744-6198.1987.tb00794.x

Zuzelo, P.R. (2007). Exploring the moral distress of registered nurses. *Nursing Ethics, 14*, 344–359. doi:10.1177/0969733007075870

CHAPTER 9

Ethics Consultation and Education

Karen Iseminger, PhD, ANP-BC, FNP, Courtney Buratto, MSN, FNP-C, OCN®, and Susan Storey, PhD, RN, AOCNS®

Introduction

Prior chapters of this publication have provided guidance to navigate through common ethically rich situations within oncology nursing, such as end-of-life issues, clinical trials, and the everyday oncology nurse experience. This final chapter offers information about the use of ethics consultation and education to address previously identified issues. An algorithm for initiating formal ethics consultation is included, and specific educational strategies for nurses are proposed. The role of the advanced practice nurse (APN), specifically the clinical nurse specialist (CNS) and nurse practitioner (NP), in ethics consultation and education is explored. A case study and an exemplar from the University of Texas MD Anderson Cancer Center are used to emphasize the value of these roles as ethics resources.

Empowering nurses to perform the duties of moral agents related to patient outcomes is challenging in the specialty of oncology. The philosophical term *agent* means "one who performs an act or action" (Thiroux, 2001, p. 523), and *morality* refers to "how humans relate to or treat one another in order to promote mutual welfare, growth, and meaning while striving for good over bad and right over wrong" (Thiroux, 2001, p. 528). Rosenstand (2006) combined these definitions and described the moral agent as "a person capable of *reflecting* on a moral problem and *acting* [emphasis added] on his or her decision" (p. 706). Rodney, Doane, Storch, and Varcoe (2006) indicated that moral agency is enacted through relationships and is nurses' professional responsibility. Moral agency *formation* is influenced by all life experiences. Formation is a distinctive aspect of human development that references virtue and the "soul" of nursing. According to Palmer (2004), *formation* is "soul work done in community" that flows from the belief that individuals are born with souls in perfect form and these souls "never stop calling us back to our birthright integrity" (pp. 57–58). Formative soul work requires acknowledgment and attentiveness if the nurse is to flourish as a moral agent.

Building on these definitions, *moral agency formation* in this chapter is considered in a new model that depicts awareness, contemplation, and courage to act within nursing endeavors. In addition to understanding what it means to be moral agents, nurses need to be aware of the abundance of ethics resources at their disposal. A three-pronged approach to resource awareness is proposed that includes ethics consultation, ethics education, and APN support. This chapter aims to empower oncology nurses by encouraging access to ethics consultation and resources, including the APN.

How the Cancer Experience Generates Ethical Concerns

A cancer diagnosis often evokes feelings of distress related to vulnerability and powerlessness. The National Comprehensive Cancer Network® (NCCN®) defined cancer-related distress as

> a multifactorial unpleasant emotional experience of a psychological (i.e., cognitive, behavioral, emotional), social, and/ or spiritual nature that may interfere with the ability to cope effectively with cancer, its physical symptoms, and its treatment. Distress extends along a continuum, ranging from common normal feelings of vulnerability, sadness, and fears to problems that can become disabling, such as depression, anxiety, panic, social isolation, and existential and spiritual crisis. (NCCN, 2015, p. DIS-2)

Many ethical dilemmas in cancer care are the direct result of the impingement on quality of life and loss of full autonomy that was available to the patient prior to diagnosis. Thus, the insult to one's identity often causes the patient to struggle with compromised self-determination, which is a critical feature of many ethical dilemmas. Because patients may be disempowered by their illness, they may be unable to share the depth of these concerns sufficiently with their physician. Therefore, nurses must acknowledge and appreciate the essential nature of the patient's experience to the greatest extent possible.

Shumaker, Anderson, and Czajkowski (1990) asserted that the quality-of-life perspective includes cognitive, social, physical, emotional, personal productivity, and intimacy dimensions. As early as the 1980s, cancer scientists recognized quality of life as a serious concern and began studying its relevance to the cancer experience. All patients experience some level of distress associated with the diagnosis and treatment of cancer (NCCN, 2015). Existential questions of angst, meaning of life, dread, and facing one's mortality also concern patients during the cancer experience. Patients receiving cancer treatment suffer physical and psychological symptoms that influence their ability to perform activities that bring value to their life.

As with any complex healthcare decision, there are times in oncology nurses' practice when they find it difficult to know the right thing to do. When one is dealing with difficult decisions, the knowledge and reflection of others can aid in the resolution of these concerns. In the ideal healthcare environment, nurses should be able to access expert resources for guidance. Nurses should be able to autonomously request a consult with the ethicist or a member of the ethics committee, or choose to discuss the issue with other available resources. (Note: Throughout this chapter, when the term *ethicist* is used, those from facilities that do not have a designated ethicist can substitute the term with *member of an ethics team or committee*.) Nurses also should be authorized to call an ethics consult if requested by patients, family members, or physicians.

Nursing's Unique Role in Addressing Ethical Concerns

Nurses are often first-line clinicians and are well suited to recognize, acknowledge, and address ethical issues in patient situations. These skills represent *ethical awareness*, defined as the ability to recognize ethical tension, understand the patient as being vulnerable, and appreciate the implications of decisions made on behalf of the individual (Lützén, Dahlqvist, Eriksson, & Norberg, 2006). In addition, nurses have a unique role in preventing ethical dilemmas. *Preventive ethics*, defined as "activities performed by an individual or group on behalf of a health care organization to identify, prioritize, and address systemic ethics issues" (Fox, Bottrell, Foglia, & Stoeckle, n.d., p. ii), may encourage ethical problem solving at the point of care. A preventive approach may thwart nurses' distress by de-escalating an ethical dilemma.

The physical nearness inherent in the nurse–patient relationship is central to the discipline of nursing and its moral ideals. In addition to the nurse being physically close to the patient, active listening skills increase sensitivity to ethical concerns. Coulehan et al. (2001) advocated that nurse clinicians focus on patients' stories in a way that fosters a fuller account of their experiences, thereby augmenting nurses' awareness of previously unspoken areas of concern. As nurses develop moral sensitivity, their ethical awareness is heightened, and they may better advocate for their patients. Iseminger (2010) approached advocacy (i.e., the moral courage to act) from a broad perspective ranging from nurses' responsibility for creating a therapeutic milieu to nursing leadership and administration, nursing education, and integration of foundational concepts requisite to understanding moral courage.

When the nurse is truly present with the patient, the groundwork is laid for a nurse–patient relationship that improves outcomes. Nursing presence builds trust and cultivates open communication, both of which are vital to effective symptom management and adherence to therapeutic goals. Through exercise of the nurse's clinical expertise, interpersonal skills, and presence, the therapeutic relationship and ethical decision making are improved. Peter and Liaschenko (2004) noted that proximity of the nurse to the patient with cancer leads to understanding and participating in cancer-related dilemmas. Thus, enhanced formation of the nurse's moral agency by means of awareness, contemplation, and courage to act is critical for empathic ethical discernment of these dilemmas.

Nurse as Moral Agent Formation Models

Two models introduced in this section illustrate a path of moral agency formation for the oncology nurse. These models put forward the introspective and relational process that is dynamic and nonsequential. The nurse as moral agent (NAMA) formation models hold that moral agency is fluid and can be formed by education, experiences, reflective practices, and clinical concern (e.g., caring for a dying patient for the first time). The first model describes ethics education, experiences with ethics consultation, and involvement and support of the APN within the context of an organizational moral milieu (see Figure 9-1). Bidirectional arrows demonstrate reciprocal relationships that sharpen the understanding of and interaction with shared experience and heighten trust within the moral milieu. LaSala and Bjarnason (2010) discussed organizational factors that stimulate moral courage. Organizations can develop their mission, vision, and values in a way that actualizes moral courage, which is essential for a therapeutic organizational milieu. Features of a therapeutic organizational milieu include transparency, a nonpunitive response to inquiry, and leadership approachability.

The second model guides nurses' individual journeys toward enhanced moral agency through increasing awareness of ethical issues, contemplation, and development of moral courage (see Figure 9-2). Nurses frequently experience their personal and professional "ideal values" being impacted by real-world constraints. For example, Tishelman et al. (2004) found that nurses' ideal values were constrained by actual clinical situations, causing internal conflict. Conquering negative emotions, which are frequently triggered by ethical dilemmas (e.g., apathy, frustration, fear), and finding courage to act demand formative growth depicted by the models. Nursing presence facilitates the relational knowledge necessary to achieve NAMA formation (Iseminger, Levitt, & Kirk, 2009).

Morally sensitive responses to a present concern can be developed by reflecting on nuances in patient care. Contemplative moral agents seek additional information about issues (e.g., potential power differences and the patient's level of understand-

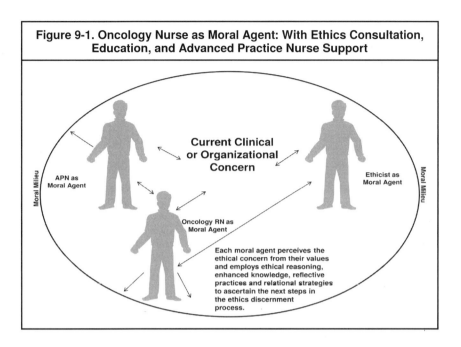

Figure 9-1. Oncology Nurse as Moral Agent: With Ethics Consultation, Education, and Advanced Practice Nurse Support

ing of medical interventions) and then act in ethically appropriate ways. The American Society for Bioethics and Humanities (ASBH, 2011) listed recommended attributes, attitudes, and behavioral competencies for NAMA formation. Ethics is not merely a prescriptive endeavor; it must end in specific ethically appropriate actions toward people in current real-time clinical or organizational situations.

Ethics Consultation as a Resource

Ethical decision making is fundamental to nursing practice and patient care. The Joint Commission (2012), an accrediting body for healthcare organizations in the United States, requires hospitals to establish committees or consultation services to address ethical dilemmas that arise in practice. According to the American Nurses Credentialing Center (ANCC), hospitals that seek Magnet® designation place strong emphasis on ethics as an integral component of quality nursing practices. The Magnet Recognition Program® distinguishes healthcare organizations for quality patient care, nursing excellence, and innovations in professional nursing practice (ANCC, 2013). Magnet organizations are required to demonstrate nurses' adherence to a code of ethics for nurses as established by the American Nurses Association (ANA, 2015) and the International Council of Nurses (ICN, 2012). These organizations support the philosophy that nurses should have a prominent voice regarding ethical issues.

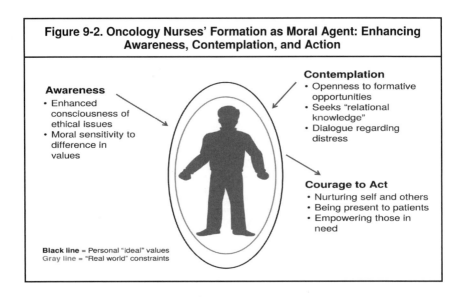

Figure 9-2. Oncology Nurses' Formation as Moral Agent: Enhancing Awareness, Contemplation, and Action

Contemplation
• Openness to formative opportunities
• Seeks "relational knowledge"
• Dialogue regarding distress

Awareness
• Enhanced consciousness of ethical issues
• Moral sensitivity to difference in values

Courage to Act
• Nurturing self and others
• Being present to patients
• Empowering those in need

Black line = Personal "ideal" values
Gray line = "Real world" constraints

Healthcare ethics consultation is a set of services provided by an individual or group in response to questions from patients, patients' families, surrogates, healthcare professionals, or other involved parties who seek to resolve uncertainty or conflict regarding value-laden concerns that emerge in health care (ASBH, 2011). Fletcher and Mosely (2003) asserted that the central purpose of ethics consultation is to improve the process and outcome of patient care by helping to identify, analyze, and resolve ethical problems. The ethics team frequently provides general ethics education and preventive ethics programs and participates in policy development.

A representative list of potential moral issues that may require the expertise of the ethicist or ethics committee includes moral distress in the patient, family, or healthcare provider; allocation of scarce resources; benefit/burden analysis in care options; consideration of the patient's best interests; confidentiality; religious or cultural values; decision-making capacity; end-of-life care (balancing curative treatment with palliative care); informed consent; non–medically indicated care; substituted judgment; treatment refusal; withdrawing or withholding treatment; autonomy; and the need for boundaries in patient care. Figures 9-3 and 9-4 demonstrate the categories of oncology-specific ethics consults at two demographically unique facilities. These data offer examples of ethics consultation issues from St. Vincent Health (compiled data from 17 Catholic healthcare facilities in Indiana) and the University of Texas MD Anderson Cancer Center, a comprehensive, oncology-specific hospital with one primary location in southeastern Texas. Shuman et al. (2013) also provided an excellent discussion about the data on oncology-related ethics consultation at Memorial Sloan Kettering Cancer Center, a leading comprehensive cancer hospital

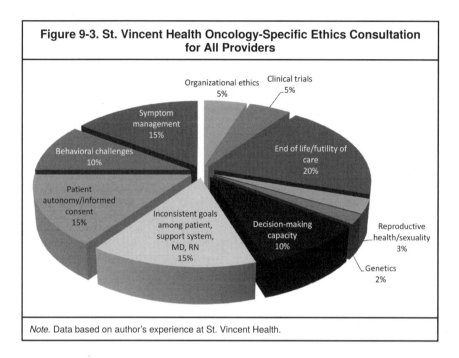

Figure 9-3. St. Vincent Health Oncology-Specific Ethics Consultation for All Providers

Organizational ethics 5%
Clinical trials 5%
Symptom management 15%
Behavioral challenges 10%
Patient autonomy/informed consent 15%
Inconsistent goals among patient, support system, MD, RN 15%
End of life/futility of care 20%
Decision-making capacity 10%
Reproductive health/sexuality 3%
Genetics 2%

Note. Data based on author's experience at St. Vincent Health.

in New York. Although the findings vary, all three organizations reported frequent consultation in the areas of end-of-life issues and perceived medical futility, inconsistent goals of care, patient autonomy, and surrogate decision making. Shuman et al. (2003) described a partial explanation for variations in the stated reasons for the ethics consult: "As those familiar with ethics consultation will invariably attest, the reason for consultation depends on one's point of view and may be perceived quite differently by the involved clinician, patient/family, and ethics consultant. . . . A large part of the ethics consultation process involves identifying the real issue at hand" (p. 244).

Additionally, just as individuals perceive ethical dilemmas differently, organizational mission and philosophy may influence conflicting perspectives among reporting entities. Institutions may hold different priorities based on factors such as size (rural versus tertiary), amount of research, presence of medical education, predominant cultures in the community, and faith-based versus secular values. To that end, John Paul Slosar, vice president of ethics at Ascension Health in St. Louis, Missouri, described several distinctive features of Catholic healthcare ethics.

> Catholic ethics is committed to following the *Ethical and Religious Directives for Catholic Health Care Services,* which emphasize our identity with the church and its concern for the body, mind, and spirit of all involved. While we do honor patient autonomy, we do so within a context of human dignity, pallia-

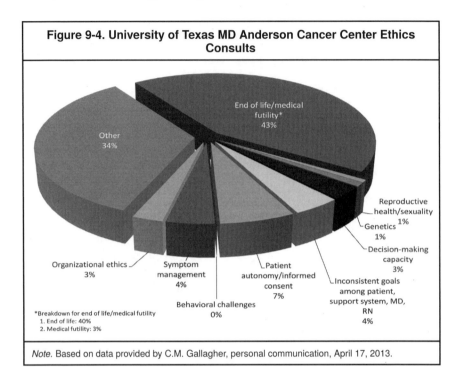

Figure 9-4. University of Texas MD Anderson Cancer Center Ethics Consults

Note. Based on data provided by C.M. Gallagher, personal communication, April 17, 2013.

tive care, and social justice. Some of our consults in the oncology setting force us to balance scarce resources regarding cost considerations with our commitment to charity care. However, the vast majority of our consults involve variations regarding treatment goals and how to best navigate when physicians and families disagree. (J.P. Slosar, personal communication, June 12, 2013)

Thus, although oncology-specific ethics consultation issues vary among individuals and organizations, there are indeed more similarities than differences. Often, what seems to be a disagreement about ethical issues arises because of problems in communication.

Many consults involve urgent decisions regarding end-of-life issues, many of which are related to disagreement between caregivers and families regarding cardiopulmonary resuscitation and other elements of "care at all costs." Generally speaking, health care should be judicious in using medical advances toward "reasonably certain" therapeutic goals. Care should be exercised to avoid exploiting extensive technology to prolong life only to appease families who refuse to acknowledge the inevitable death of their loved one. The situation is even more complicated in pediatric cancer units where clinicians are challenged to decide how much technologic support to provide to society's youngest members who have not had the opportunity to live, who cannot speak for themselves, and for whom prognostication is difficult.

Contemporary Approaches to Ethics Consultation

Oncology nurses relate many personal experiences that cause them to question whether their patients are receiving situation-specific, value-based care. An algorithm for clinical ethics consultation used by a large Midwestern facility is offered as an example of how to address nurses' concerns (see Figure 9-5). The algorithm is intended to be used as a tool for healthcare providers when trying to determine the right thing to do and is available to all employees as a web-based policy found on the organization's intranet.

Nurses are encouraged to seek additional understanding and resolution by discussing the matter with clinical leadership, APNs, unit or department managers, attending physicians, chaplains, or other members of the healthcare team. If the conflict is unresolved within the family or on the nursing unit, the ethicist may assist in facilitating communication and resolution of the issue. Supportive organizational leadership encourages nurses to raise questions and seek guidance, clarification, and solutions to any ethical concerns they may have. Furthermore, the ethics team fosters and facilitates debriefing of clinical situations that have produced significant moral angst. Such opportunities help to lessen negative emotional responses and create a safe environment to discuss feelings about challenging situations. Effective organizations openly communicate the method for contacting an ethics resource.

A primary goal for ethics consultants is to become acquainted with the stakeholders (patient, family, physicians, and other clinicians) involved in the ethical dilemma. This is achieved by being present to notice nuances and contextualization of their experiences that they might not be able or willing to express via direct verbal communication. In so doing, the consultant can share in the lived experience of the distressed moral agent. Gadow (1999) described this "relational knowledge" as a vital component of ethical discernment. Wright and Brajtman (2011) suggested the following.

> Nursing's distinct perspective on the moral matters of health care stem not from any privileged vantage point but rather from knowledge developed through the daily activities of nursing practice. . . . In everyday clinical care, nurses cultivate ethical knowledge of at least two forms: (1) relational knowledge and (2) embodied knowledge. (p. 20)

Gadow (1999) emphasized that relational ethics should replace detached reason. Relational ethics is a method of addressing uncertainty or conflict that stems from value-laden issues that emerge in the healthcare setting. The requirement that ethics consultation should be relationally based also correlates with the ASBH (2011) chapter "Character and Ethics Consultation."

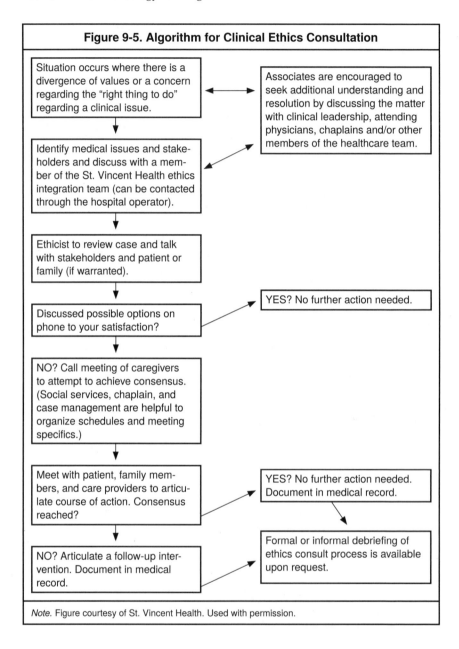

Figure 9-5. Algorithm for Clinical Ethics Consultation

Situation occurs where there is a divergence of values or a concern regarding the "right thing to do" regarding a clinical issue.

Associates are encouraged to seek additional understanding and resolution by discussing the matter with clinical leadership, attending physicians, chaplains and/or other members of the healthcare team.

Identify medical issues and stake-holders and discuss with a member of the St. Vincent Health ethics integration team (can be contacted through the hospital operator).

Ethicist to review case and talk with stakeholders and patient or family (if warranted).

Discussed possible options on phone to your satisfaction?

YES? No further action needed.

NO? Call meeting of caregivers to attempt to achieve consensus. (Social services, chaplain, and case management are helpful to organize schedules and meeting specifics.)

Meet with patient, family members, and care providers to articulate course of action. Consensus reached?

YES? No further action needed. Document in medical record.

Formal or informal debriefing of ethics consult process is available upon request.

NO? Articulate a follow-up intervention. Document in medical record.

Note. Figure courtesy of St. Vincent Health. Used with permission.

Exemplary attributes of the relationally oriented moral agent are listed in Table 9-1 with actions that describe the aptitude of each trait.

Walker's (1993) discussion on "keeping moral space open" offered a new vision of ethics consultation. She suggested rethinking the ethics consultant as a spe-

Table 9-1. Attributes of Moral Agents	
Attributes	**Actions**
Tolerance, patience, and compassion	Enable listening well and communication of interest, respect, support, and empathy.
Honesty, forthrightness, and self-knowledge	Prevent manipulative use of information and create an atmosphere of trust.
Courage	Promote effective communication of all parties.
Prudence and humility	Inform behavior when rash decisions are considered and prevent overstepping the bounds of role in consultation.
Leadership	Represent ethics within institution, support strategic planning for consultation, and strive for improvement in ethics knowledge, skills, and practice.
Integrity	Enable pursuit of a range of options ethically required even when doing otherwise might be more convenient.

Note. Based on information from American Society for Bioethics and Humanities, 2011.

cial sort of teacher whose job is to role model analysis and reflection, describing the ethicist as a type of architect who creates moral space for the requisite dialogue for relational knowledge to occur. She also advocated that these open moral spaces be undergirded by many of the same character qualities identified in the ASBH competencies. Open moral spaces are an integral part of the moral milieu that allows the NAMA to flourish.

In addition to moral dilemma resolution, other interventions the ethicist may use to support nurses who work in highly stress-producing areas involve strategies to enhance preventive ethics, a primary focal point of the ethicist. As the ethicist identifies clinical patterns and assists in developing alternative practices, then perhaps another "futility" consult can be avoided. Use of the humanities (e.g., health-related films, art, and literature) in the clinical area assists in influencing deficient practitioner patterns by enhancing empathy, self-assessment, and sensitivity to moral issues (Hawkins & Chandler-McEntyre, 2000). Several authors specifically recommended passage meditation, mindful practice formation, and mindful meditation (Davies, 2008; Frankel, Eddins-Folensbee, & Inui, 2011; Oman, Hedberg, & Thoresen, 2006). These interventions have been demonstrated to be effective as strategies to reduce stress and enhance mental health (Oman et al., 2006). Innovative educational methods to disseminate these contemporary strategies are described, in part, in the following section on ethics education.

Ethics Education

Nurses demonstrate competence of many tangible psychomotor skills by objective measurement. Such measurements, however, are not effective for determining ability to act as a moral agent. There is no prescription for the amount of ethics education needed to make a nurse ethically minded. The following section offers recommendations for how best to educate nurses about ethics and the role it plays in practice. Perhaps the most crucial step is to expose nursing students to practice scenarios in which they must identify ethical dilemmas and discuss how to best resolve them.

Formal Undergraduate Ethics Education

Ethics instruction beginning at the onset of nursing education is imperative to prepare nurses for entry into a challenging moral environment. To that end, primary commitment to the patient, patient advocacy, preservation of integrity and moral self-respect, and promotion of moral agency by example are included in the *Code of Ethics for Nurses* (ANA, 2015). Ethics is an integral part of nursing practice and involves respect and advocacy for the rights and needs of patients regardless of setting. The American Association of Colleges of Nursing (AACN, 2008) asserted that "honesty and acting ethically are two key elements of professional behavior, which have a major impact on patient safety" (p. 27). Although these standards exist, there are no specific requirements regarding the amount of content or method of instruction, or metrics to evaluate mastery of concepts and their clinical application.

Abstract ethics concepts require active engagement of the learner as well as opportunities for application. Ethics content warrants exploration of moral dilemmas and reflective practice about how to resolve ethical distress. Facing moral dilemmas is an inevitable part of nursing practice, especially in the specialty of oncology where patient acuity and complex healthcare decision making naturally create challenging scenarios. Nurses must envision themselves in these situations and reflect on what it means to have moral courage and moral agency when acting on behalf of their patients. Using these terms to impart ethics understanding enables the nurse to integrate principles into practice and embody moral agency.

Current practices in teaching ethics concepts vary, and a review of the literature offers no definitive method for achieving optimal outcomes. Therefore, the authors suggest that a stand-alone ethics course be required along with an integrative approach to reiterate concepts. An ethics course near the beginning of the nursing curriculum offers the greatest impact and should cover ethical principles and provide a foundation for ethics comprehension (Park, Kjervik, Crandell, & Oermann, 2012). Reflective writing assignments and group discussion about case scenarios should be used to enhance the application of concepts to moral agency formation. Revisiting ethics in subsequent semesters promotes contemplation of ethical concepts as nursing knowledge expands, allowing students to use resources they may employ in the real world to identify and resolve ethical dilemmas in their practice. By revisiting ethics each semester, students will have their own clinical examples to use as a basis for discussion. Park et al. (2012) found that each hour of ethics content increased critical-thinking ability and moral reasoning of nursing students; therefore, the amount of exposure is significant. Scholastic ethics education produced nurses who were more confident in moral judgment and more prone to use ethics resources, whereas nurses who infrequently used consultation services had little to no ethics training and felt unqualified (Park et al., 2012). When nurses lacked a framework within which to understand and solve dilemmas, they were more likely to experience moral distress and compassion fatigue (Grady et al., 2008).

Informal Ethics Education

Informal ethics education can take the form of courses or conferences offered by hospitals or organizations, online modules, facilitated ethics conversations, and formative literature programs with or without a narrative component (see Table 9-2). Nurse colleagues and mentors are also sources of ethics education. For example, oncology nurses in one study indicated that other nurses and CNSs are the most helpful roles to support coping (Raines, 2000).

Frequently, ethics consults are generated not solely by the medical aspects of a patient's case but instead because of a patient and family situation that causes angst. Another way in which nurses can be prepared to address these types of conditions is through the study of the medical humanities, which addresses nonphysical aspects of illness such as wellness, mortality, spirituality, and personal values. Questions that arise related to this approach include what makes us human, what defines us as individuals, how can we reconcile the needs of the individual with the needs of the community, what gives meaning to our lives, and what constitutes the good life (Dittrich, 2003).

Evans (2002) suggested that exposing students to medical humanities would, among other things, encourage them to identify, explore, develop, and sustain their own personal values. Literature provides opportunities for exploration that many people do not experience in real life. If clinicians can better relate to patients and other healthcare workers on a spiritual level, then healthcare institutions will become more humane places of healing.

Relevant to formation of the nurse as moral agent, Emily S. Beckman, assistant clinical professor of medical humanities at Indiana University–Purdue University Indianapolis, emphasized improving empathy in medical students through use of literature as a teaching method.

> The content of our medical humanities classes is perfectly suited for nurses. Nurses offer great insight during our discussions and are generally quite empathetic. In fact, they are often

the first to recognize a lack of empathy/compassion in many of our readings. It seems that what they want or need to know is how to better respond when empathy is lacking in the clinical situation. Our facilitated discussions seem to shed light on their quest for moral courage. (E.S. Beckman, personal communication, April 19, 2013)

Nurses have autonomy and accountability for patient outcomes; therefore, ethics is an innate component to these role characteristics. In order to advocate

	Table 9-2. Ethics Resources	
Organization	**Offerings**	**Website**
American Nurses Association	• *Code of Ethics for Nurses* • Center for Ethics and Human Rights • Moral Courage and Distress	www.nursingworld.org
International Council of Nurses	• *The ICN Code of Ethics for Nurses*	www.icn.ch/about-icn/code-of-ethics-for-nurses
Lippincott's NursingCenter	• Resources for dealing with end-of-life issues, personal moral dilemmas • Review of ethical principles, professional values, and legal issues	www.nursingcenter.com
National Center for Ethics in Health Care	• Educational programs • Ethics pocket cards	www.ethics.va.gov/index.asp
Oncology Nursing Society	• Position statements • *Ethics in Oncology Nursing*	www.ons.org
Facility-based	• Ethics committees/ethicists • Seminars • Advanced practice nurses	Consult institution website or contact management or human resources.
Publications	• *American Journal of Bioethics* • *American Journal of Nursing* • *Health Care Ethics USA* • *Nursing Ethics*	www.bioethics.net http://journals.lww.com/ajnonline/pages/default.aspx www.chausa.org/publications/health-care-ethics-usa http://nej.sagepub.com

for patients, nurses must understand patient goals and ensure alignment with the plan of care. Accordingly, continuing education requirements for nurses should include ethics content (Park, 2009).

Online ethics resources abound, and many hospitals have their own resources. Furthermore, nurses can initiate informal ethics discussions or unscheduled conversations that provide support and can organize an ethics journal club or library to keep resources readily available to the unit (Raines, 2000).

In summary, the benefits of quality ethics education include increased confidence in moral judgment and use of ethics resources (Grady et al., 2008). Nurses who have received adequate education should be able to identify scenarios that may lead to moral distress in order to intervene accordingly. Decreased compassion fatigue and enhanced patient experience are outcomes of the responsible ethics education described in this chapter.

Enhanced Access Through Advanced Practice Nursing

Health care is in the throes of constant transition, which impacts the ethical questions that nurses face daily. APNs are well positioned to identify and address ethical issues in practice by using an interdisciplinary approach (Rodney et al., 2006). As described by Salyer and Frazelle (2014), "Advanced practice nursing includes specialization but goes beyond it; it involves expansion, which legitimizes role autonomy, and advancement, characterized by the integration of a broad range of theoretical, research-based, and practical knowledge" (p. 113). For the purpose of this chapter, *APN* refers to both the CNS and NP roles as they relate to ethics consultation and education.

APN practice is founded on core knowledge of ethics and requires commitment to lifelong learning about ethical issues to address the discord created by societal issues and technologic advancements (Hamric & Delgado, 2014). Rapid changes in health care and science require APNs to anticipate potential ethical concerns. Nurses in oncology settings have greater exposure to ethical situations than those who work in other areas of patient care (Cohen & Erickson, 2006); therefore, the role of the APN as an oncology ethics resource is pivotal. The principle of subsidiarity purports that individuals who are the closest and most pivotal to the ethical dilemma should have a voice in its resolution. Accordingly, APNs are in a unique position to assist nurses, as the bedside approach to ethics resolution is quicker, closer, and often more effective than other means of resolving ethical issues. This ensures that decisions are made at the most appropriate level without the encumbrance of delaying action while those closest to the patient defer to higher authorities or committees.

The role of APNs and the requirement that their education include greater comprehension and expertise in healthcare ethics facilitate real-time ethics consultation. Professional organizations such as the Oncology Nursing Society

(ONS) have clearly articulated through competency statements their expectations of the APN as the role relates to ethical practices and activities (ONS, 2007, 2008). Ethical decision making and conduct have been identified as essential characteristics for influential and effective APN practice (Bingle & Davidson, 2014; National Clinical Nurse Specialist Competency Task Force, 2010). APN ethical conduct includes fostering autonomy and truth telling; advocacy for patients, families, and other nurses; and facilitating dignity with end-of-life issues across the continuum of care (National Association of Clinical Nurse Specialists, 2004; ONS, 2008).

Cassells, Jenkins, Lea, Calzone, and Johnson (2003) studied oncology nurses and concluded that although the number of ethical issues they experienced in daily practice had increased, nurses perceived they were minimally prepared to address and resolve them. Nurses are often unaware or unsure of how to use ethical theories to inform their actions and decisions. APNs have the knowledge and ability to integrate the tenets of theory and research into daily practice and guide patients and the healthcare team through decision making from which strategies for resolution are generated.

NPs and CNSs have different scopes of practice, which provide unique skill sets available to nursing. The ethics competencies of the NP are to integrate ethical principles into decision making, evaluate the ethical consequences of decisions, and apply ethically sound solutions to complex issues (National Organization of Nurse Practitioner Faculties, 2012). Iseminger (2000) asserted that all NP students have the willingness and knowledge to perceive to the greatest extent possible the essential nature of their patients' experiences. One way to accomplish this goal is via a quality-of-life perspective, which is particularly relevant for clinical decision making. NPs understand the nurses' moral responsibilities and the medical diagnosis and treatment plan and are therefore able to thwart distress through enhanced communication of goals, demonstrating preventive ethics.

ONS identified oncology CNSs as expert clinicians who provide care and advocacy to patients with cancer and their families across the continuum of care (ONS, 2008). CNS behaviors associated with knowledge of ethics and decision making are moral agency, advocacy, identification, articulation, and action related to ethical concerns at the patient, family, healthcare provider, system, community, and public policy levels (McClelland, McCoy, & Burson, 2013). An important role of the CNS is interaction with nurses and patients through interdisciplinary rounds. Rounds enable CNSs to identify ethical issues, implement preventive ethics, and facilitate interdisciplinary problem-solving skills and teamwork. CNSs identify patient needs and implement theory and evidence-based interventions into daily patient care to ensure quality and safety. They advance nursing practice by mentoring nurses and can provide informal ethics education through real-time discussions on the unit with patients, family members, nurses, or other healthcare team members. CNSs also can organize informal educational opportunities related to ethics, such as workshops, in-services, and lunch-and-learn programs. Additionally, they can facilitate debriefing sessions, which provide an opportunity to learn from experience and inform future actions in a nonthreatening environment.

APNs serve as role models and resources for the implementation of ethical practice in the clinical setting. The accessibility of an APN lends itself to being a resource for staff nurses in need of consultation. The clinical demands and high acuity of patients in the oncology setting may be a deterrent to proceeding with a formal ethics consultation in times of moral distress. The APN may function as an ethics triage point by evaluating whether resolution can be reached without a formal ethics consultation.

Advanced Practice Nurse Influence on the Moral Milieu

In addition to the application of knowledge in the clinical setting, APNs must be aware of their personal moral agency and values to promote consistent behavior in the clinical setting. This allows the APN to develop boundaries that prevent undue influence over the outcome for those involved in the ethical situation (Hamric & Delgado, 2014). Assessment of the moral milieu on a unit occurs through direct interaction with patients and families, nurses, and other members of the healthcare team. Georges and Grypdonck (2002) suggested that nurses find it easier to identify significant ethical issues (e.g., euthanasia) than to articulate those ethical tensions and issues within their everyday encounters. High patient acuity and increased demands on nurses often require their focus to be on tasks and routines surrounding patient care. When nurses become mired in the routine, it impedes their ability and sensitivity to recognize the ethical issues at hand. This "routinization of the world" can create a detrimental milieu in which nurses do not realize they are facing an ethical situation (Chamblis, 1996). APNs can bring such situations to the attention of the healthcare team and work to address the system issues that perpetuate it.

Recognition of an ethical situation is highly subjective and dependent on the nurse's unique set of beliefs and attitudes. The degree to which the ethical issue becomes problematic will vary from nurse to nurse (Cohen & Erickson, 2006). Nurses involved in direct patient care often feel powerless to address ethical issues. As respected members of the healthcare team, APNs can flatten the hierarchical organizational relationships that exist among healthcare team members. They also can lead interdisciplinary discussions among team members to clarify the plan of care and recognize ethical issues as they arise. Armed with advanced communication skills and ability to establish a nonthreatening, nonjudgmental atmosphere, APNs promote mutual respect, open communication, and transparency among healthcare team members.

Case Study

Beatrice Duffy is a 47-year-old woman with advanced lung cancer. She is admitted for respiratory distress and changes in level of consciousness related to brain metastasis. The oncologist proposes more chemotherapy, but Ms. Duffy tells her sister and the nurse that she is "tired of living this way" and wants to stop treatment. She consents to treatment, however, under pressure from her mother. As Ms. Duffy's condition deteriorates, her mother insists that the chemotherapy be administered. The nurse informs the physician of Ms. Duffy's conflicting messages about the desire to continue chemotherapy and requests that a palliative care referral be made. The physician responds that no palliative care consult is needed and requests that chemotherapy be initiated promptly.

Ms. Duffy's condition continues to deteriorate, and the nurse pages the physician to inform him of the patient's continued decline in status, discuss the patient's code status, and express discomfort with administering chemotherapy. The mother is distraught that chemotherapy is held as she is still hoping that the treatment will cure her daughter. While awaiting a call back from the physician, the rapid response team is summoned, and upon evaluation, the rapid response physician orders a "no code" status. Ms. Duffy dies shortly thereafter.

Discussion

In this situation, the bedside nurse would have benefited from clinical resources and a culture that encouraged moral courage to ask questions and have concerns validated. An oncology-certified NP or CNS available to the inpatient unit, for example, could efficiently perform a more thorough assessment and act as a resource for the nurse. The NP could validate and explore the nurse's findings and act as a moral agent to recognize the nurse's distress and help to make a clinical decision (i.e., preventive ethics). The NP could relay findings to the physicians with recommendations about appropriateness of the plan of care or need for diagnostics, referrals, and treatment. Other resources that could be available to the nurse in this scenario are looking to the nurse manager for direction and arranging a formal ethics consultation to discuss best practice options in future similar scenarios.

Ethical Decision-Making Process

As portrayed in the case study, the nurse can choose to seek additional input from colleagues when raising an ethical concern. Other colleagues, including nurses, the APN, and the respiratory therapist; consultation with the palliative care team; or consultation with the ethics team can support the nurse to follow the six steps of the ethical decision-making process described by Purtilo and Doherty (2011). These steps are an appropriate process for all oncology nurses to learn and use.

Step 1: Gather information. Information gathering is necessary to understand the complexity of the issue and the conflicting points of view. A review of the medical record and discussions with the nurse, patient, family members, and oncologist provide the contextual perspective of each key stakeholder. The nurse identifies key pieces of information that were poorly understood, such as the patient's prognosis, the patient's desire to abstain from further treatment, and the mother's insistence on additional treatment.

Step 2: Identify the type of ethical problem. Hamric and Delgado (2014) discussed three types of ethical problems: moral dilemmas, moral uncertainty, and moral distress. In the case study, each of these types of problems occurs simultaneously. Each person is competing for control: the patient desires to stop treatment, the patient's mother assumes decision-making duties, the oncologist refuses to make referrals for available resources, and the nurse attempts to advocate for the patient's wishes. A complex ethical dilemma exists because of the opposing desires of the physician, nurse, family, and patient. Moral distress occurs because stakeholders feel they are unable to carry out the course of action they believe is right.

A colleague in a mediator position, such as an oncology CNS, can act as an objective resource to identify the ethical problem. By interacting with stakeholders, the CNS validates individual concerns, recognizes angst, and empowers articulation of the ethical problem from all perspectives. Consultation with the ethicist on the team may be necessary to articulate particularly complex ethical problems.

Step 3: Use ethical theories or approaches to analyze the problem. Oncology CNSs are equipped with advanced problem-solving skills and can establish working relationships with resources that supplement their ability to resolve ethical problems. Ideally, the CNS employs these resources at the outset of ethical dilemma identification to prevent escalation. The perceptive CNS realizes that the intensity of the situation warrants additional resources such as a formal ethics consultation to facilitate resolution.

Through consultation, the advanced knowledge of ethicists situates them as excellent resources to assist nurses in using ethical theories and principles to evaluate clinical issues and avert inappropriate outcomes and further nurse distress. In the case of a patient who is dying, the participants will most likely struggle with balancing deontological ethics (the duty of the nurse to be a spokesperson for the patient) with the utilitarian approach (acquiescing to the more powerful mother and physician). During the deliberation, the ethicist is likely to use virtue-based theories of caring and feminist ethics. The feminist ethics concern for the marginalized patient is particularly apt when patients feel disempowered by illness and possess diminished personal productivity capabilities. Moreover, relation-based ethics assists the ethicist to know the stakeholders well enough to mediate the dilemma by honoring individuals' values. Ultimately, adherence to ANA's *Code of Ethics for Nurses* would trump other strategies because of its directive for nurses to advocate for their patients regardless of any personal consequences.

Step 4: Explore practical alternatives. Often scenarios are time-sensitive situations requiring immediate intervention. The CNS and ethicist, by quickly organizing a discussion among stakeholders, may have been able to achieve resolution. Patients and nurses often feel disadvantaged because of the imbalance of power relative to professional members of the healthcare team. The CNS and/or ethicist acting as an advocate for the patient and nurse could have mitigated the imbalance by allowing the perspective of each member to be heard. Optimally, with each perspective in mind, the ethicist acts as a liaison to communicate the patient's wishes to the family and healthcare team. Treatment side effects, the consequences of no treatment, and end-of-life issues needed to be discussed to provide a realistic picture of available options and their outcomes. In the end, treatment should only be appropriate if it is in line with the patient's goals.

Step 5: Complete the action. Moral courage is required to complete the determined plan of action. There are often repercussions for taking action to resolve difficult ethical situations, but consequences for inaction are present as well. Unpleasant encounters may occur with colleagues and the patient's family members when the nurse advocates on behalf of the patient. Moral agency requires that the situation be addressed, which, in this case, means supporting the patient's desire to decline chemotherapy while respectfully addressing the concerns of all stakeholders. The presence of the CNS and ethicist offers additional support for the patient, family, and nursing staff.

Step 6: Evaluate the action. When the situation is resolved, evaluating the action, process, and outcome is an important final step. The CNS, along with the ethicist, creates and supports opportunities for reflection and debriefing. Reflective practices allow staff to consider events, evaluate behaviors and alternatives, and develop a plan to follow in future situations (Zuzelo, 2010). Facilitation of a debriefing session by the ethicist following the case study scenario empowered the nurses involved to evaluate their feelings and actions and enhanced their confidence as moral agents. Ethical situations often are charged with emotion, and reflective practice and debriefing can enhance coping strategies for healthcare team members (Schluter, Winch, Holzhauser, & Henderson, 2008). Additionally, individual ethics consults serve as stimuli for organizational ethical discernment to improve practice and prevent future patients from facing similar dilemmas. APNs can partner with ethicists and ethics teams to discuss various provider initiatives in the organization, such as implementing guidelines and standards about professional practice issues, especially those related to advanced and end-of-life care, as illustrated in this case study. Other initiatives might include training to improve communication and interprofessional collaboration skills and clinical resources to facilitate informed consent and decision making in intensive care and end-of-life situations.

An Exemplar of Support for Oncology Nurses

The University of Texas MD Anderson Cancer Center in Houston has established an exemplary ethics program that depicts the vital role of nursing in dealing with ethical concerns. The institution's commitment to the role of nursing, as described by Colleen M. Gallagher, chief and executive director of the Section of Integrated Ethics in Cancer Care, includes nursing ethics educational programs, nursing ethics grand rounds, an "ethics corner" on the nursing website, and establishment of a Nursing Ethics Professional Action Coordinating Team. Additionally, they have created a role for a specially trained APN who is integral to the organizational team (C.M. Gallagher, personal communication, April 17, 2013).

MD Anderson Cancer Center's nursing-specific ethics endeavors were born out of the institution's clinical ethics committee's analysis of ethics consultations. The institution designed the support mechanisms listed previously to allow for more nurse involvement in addressing patient care, research, quality, and administrative ethical concerns and to provide more robust institutional recognition of the nursing role. Thus, the organizational milieu enhances nurses' moral agency formation by respecting the integral role of nursing to identify, educate, and provide resources for resolving ethical issues in the delivery of care from a nursing perspective, as these affect patients and nursing practice.

Conclusion

This chapter discussed current methods for ethics education and consultation and offered suggestions about how to improve and supplement current practices in the oncology setting. APNs can act as an ethics resource and facilitator of preventive ethics. The authors champion the notion that oncology nurses as moral agents have the opportunity to be supported during their formation by personalized resources as depicted by the NAMA models (i.e., contemporary ethics consultation, effective ethics education practices, and support by APN interventions). For institutions without an identified ethicist, mechanisms by which to address ethical dilemmas, such as an ethics committee, can be called upon. Other resources available include APNs, chaplains, social workers, leadership, and nurse colleagues. Professionals at ANA or state nurses associations also may be contacted for non-urgent dilemma resolution.

The primary goal of this chapter is for nurses to have an increased voice in ethical discernment as moral agents who have been formed by enhanced ethics awareness, compassionate contemplation, and courage to act. It is of utmost importance that this course of action would result in improved quality-of-life–oriented and ethically sensitive care for patients with cancer and their families.

Suggested Reading

American Society for Bioethics and Humanities. (2009). *Improving competencies in clinical ethics consultation: An education guide.* Glenview, IL: Author.

American Society for Bioethics and Humanities. (2011). *Core competencies for healthcare ethics consultation* (2nd ed.). Glenview, IL: Author.

These publications complement each other, as the first describes standards (access to consultation, systematic processes for responding to requests for ethics consultation, quality measures), competencies and skills (meeting facilitation, assessment, analysis skills), core knowledge (legal issues, classic ethics cases), and recommended evaluation methods (methods and tool for ethics data analysis), while the second provides detailed educational strategies such as literature review, simulation strategies, and value clarification exercises to accomplish these competencies.

Aulisio, M.P., Arnold, R.M., & Youngner, S.J. (Eds.). (2003). *Ethics consultation: From theory to practice*. Baltimore, MD: Johns Hopkins University Press.

Significant content from this text includes salient descriptions of why ethics consultation is needed and how consultation can be adapted to meet increasingly complex medical decisions and shifting healthcare environments. Moreover, it provides readers with pragmatic approaches to issues such as the relationship between character development and ethics consultation, ethics training techniques (e.g., teaching of psychotherapy skills), innovative educational programs (e.g., spontaneous problem-centered learning and/or prescribed multiday workshops), and the structure of ethics consult services (e.g., one-member ethics team versus an entire committee).

Catholic Health Association of the United States. (2014). *Striving for excellence in ethics: A resource for the Catholic health ministry* (2nd ed.). St. Louis, MO: Author.

This publication expresses what the Catholic Health Association of the United States recommends for a robust ethics service. Included in the recommendations are standards for the following categories: ethics expertise (master's versus doctoral education for clinical ethicists), ethics committees (structure regarding disciplines, skills, and expertise of committee members), consultation and advisement (ethics consultation service need for mediation skills, working knowledge of educational and religious directives), education and formation (teaching essential knowledge and information as well as strategies for influencing the organizational culture over time), policy review and development (surrogate decision-making policy, care of the poor), community outreach (connecting with public needs beyond the institution), institutional integration (ethicist as a voice in other key committees throughout the organization), and leadership support (adequate budget to meet the ethics equality standards).

References

American Association of Colleges of Nursing. (2008). *The essentials of baccalaureate education for professional nursing practice*. Retrieved from http://www.aacn.nche.edu/education-resources/bacces sentials08.pdf

American Nurses Association. (2015). *Code of ethics for nurses with interpretive statements.* Retrieved from http://www.nursingworld.org/MainMenuCategories/DocumentFault/Ethics_1CodeofEthics forNurses.html

American Nurses Credentialing Center. (2013). ANCC Magnet Recognition Program®. Retrieved from http://nursecredentialing.org/Magnet

American Society for Bioethics and Humanities. (2011). *Core competencies for healthcare ethics consultation* (2nd ed.). Glenview, IL: Author.

Bingle, J.M., & Davidson, S.B. (2014). Professional attributes in the context of emotional intelligence, ethical conduct, and citizenship of the clinical nurse specialist. In J.S. Fulton, B.L. Lyon, & K.A. Goudreau (Eds.), *Foundations of clinical nurse specialist practice* (2nd ed., pp. 17–31). New York, NY: Springer.

Cassells, J.M., Jenkins, J., Lea, D.H., Calzone, K., & Johnson, E. (2003). An ethical assessment framework for addressing global genetic issues in clinical practice. *Oncology Nursing Forum, 30,* 383–390. doi:10.1188/03.ONF.383-390

Chamblis, D.F. (1996). *Beyond caring: Hospitals, nurses, and the social organization of ethics.* Chicago, IL: University of Chicago Press.

Cohen, J.S., & Erickson, J.M. (2006). Ethical dilemmas and moral distress in oncology nursing practice. *Clinical Journal of Oncology Nursing, 10,* 775–780. doi:10.1188/06.CJON.775-780

Coulehan, J.L., Platt, F.W., Egener, B., Frankel, R., Lin, C.-T., Lown, B., & Salazar, W.H. (2001). "Let me see if I have this right . . .": Words that help build empathy. *Annals of Internal Medicine, 135,* 221–227. doi:10.7326/0003-4819-135-3-200108070-00022

Davies, W.R. (2008). Mindful meditation: Healing burnout in critical care nursing. *Holistic Nursing Practice, 22,* 32–36. doi:10.1097/01.HNP.0000306326.56955.14

Dittrich, L.R. (2003). Preface. *Academic Medicine, 78,* 951–952. doi:10.1097/00001888-200310000 -00001

Evans, M. (2002). Reflections on the humanities in medical education. *Medical Education, 36,* 508–513. doi:10.1046/j.1365-2923.2002.01225.x

Fletcher, J.C., & Mosely, K.L. (2003). The structure and process of ethics consultation services. In M.P. Aulisio, R.M. Arnold, & S.J. Youngner (Eds.), *Ethics consultation: From theory to practice* (pp. 96–117). Baltimore, MD: Johns Hopkins University Press.

Fox, E., Bottrell, M., Foglia, M.B., & Stoeckle, R. (n.d.). *Preventive ethics: Addressing ethics quality gaps on a systems level.* Retrieved from http://www.ethics.va.gov/PEprimer.pdf

Frankel, R.M., Eddins-Folensbee, F., & Inui, T.S. (2011). Crossing the patient-centered divide: Transforming health care quality through enhanced faculty development. *Academic Medicine, 86,* 445–452. doi:10.1097/ACM.0b013e31820e7e6e

Gadow, S. (1999). Relational narrative: The postmodern turn in nursing ethics. *Scholarly Inquiry for Nursing Practice, 13,* 57–70.

Georges, J.J., & Grypdonck, M. (2002). Moral problems experienced by nurses when caring for terminally ill people: A literature review. *Nursing Ethics, 9,* 155–178. doi:10.1191/0969733002ne 495oa

Grady, C., Danis, M., Soeken, K.L., O'Donnell, P., Taylor, C., Farrar, A., & Ulrich, C.M. (2008). Does ethics education influence the moral action of practicing nurses and social workers? *American Journal of Bioethics, 8*(4), 4–11. doi:10.1080/15265160802166017

Hamric, A.B., & Delgado, S.A. (2014). Ethical decision making In A.B. Hamric, J.A. Spross, & C.M. Hanson (Eds.), *Advanced practice nursing: An integrative approach* (5th ed., pp. 328–358). St. Louis, MO: Elsevier Saunders.

Hawkins, A.H., & Chandler-McEntyre, M. (Eds.). (2000). *Teaching literature and medicine.* New York, NY: Modern Language Association.

International Council of Nurses. (2012). *The ICN code of ethics for nurses.* Retrieved from http://www. icn.ch/images/stories/documents/about/icncode_english.pdf

Iseminger, K. (2000). Quality of life considerations as the foundation for decision making: An integrated program for nurse practitioner students. In K. Crabtree (Ed.), *Teaching clinical decision mak-*

ing in advanced nursing practice (pp. 37–43). Washington, DC: National Organization of Nurse Practitioner Faculties.

Iseminger, K. (2010). Overview and summary: Moral courage amid moral distress: Strategies or action. *Online Journal of Issues in Nursing, 15*(3). doi:10.3912/OJIN.Vol15No03ManOS

Iseminger, K., Levitt, F., & Kirk, L. (2009). Healing during existential moments: The "art" of nursing presence. *Nursing Clinics of North America, 44,* 447–459. doi:10.1016/j.cnur.2009.07.001

Joint Commission. (2012). *Hospital accreditation standards 2013.* Oakbrook Terrace, IL: Joint Commission Resources.

LaSala, C.A., & Bjarnason, D. (2010). Creating workplace environments that support moral courage. *Online Journal of Issues in Nursing, 15*(3). doi:10.3912/OJIN.Vol15No03Man4

Lützén, K., Dahlqvist, V., Eriksson, S., & Norberg, A. (2006). Developing the concept of moral sensitivity in health care practice. *Nursing Ethics, 13,* 187–196. doi:10.1191/0969733006ne837oa

McClelland, M., McCoy, M.A., & Burson, R. (2013). Clinical nurse specialists: Then, now, and the future of the profession. *Clinical Nurse Specialist, 27,* 96–102. doi:10.1097/NUR.0b013e3182819154

National Association of Clinical Nurse Specialists. (2004). *Statement on clinical nurse specialist practice and education* (2nd ed.). Harrisburg, PA: Author.

National Clinical Nurse Specialist Competency Task Force. (2010). *Clinical nurse specialist core competencies.* Retrieved from http://www.nacns.org/docs/CNSCoreCompetenciesBroch.pdf

National Comprehensive Cancer Network. (2015). *NCCN Clinical Practice Guidelines in Oncology (NCCN Guidelines®): Distress management* [v.3.2015]. Retrieved from http://www.nccn.org/professionals/physician_gls/pdf/distress.pdf

National Organization of Nurse Practitioner Faculties. (2012). *Nurse practitioner core competencies.* Retrieved from http://c.ymcdn.com/sites/www.nonpf.org/resource/resmgr/competencies/npcorecompetenciesfinal2012.pdf

Oman, D., Hedberg, J., & Thoresen, C.E. (2006). Passage meditation reduces perceived stress in health professionals: A randomized, controlled trial. *Journal of Consulting and Clinical Psychology, 74,* 714–719. doi:10.1037/0022-006x.74.4.714

Oncology Nursing Society. (2007). *Oncology nurse practitioner competencies.* Retrieved from https://www.ons.org/sites/default/files/npcompentencies.pdf

Oncology Nursing Society. (2008). *Oncology clinical nurse specialist competencies.* Retrieved from https://www.ons.org/sites/default/files/cnscomps.pdf

Palmer, P.J. (2004). *A hidden wholeness: The journey toward an undivided life.* San Francisco, CA: Jossey-Bass.

Park, M. (2009). The legal basis of nursing ethics education. *Journal of Nursing Law, 13,* 106–113. doi:10.1891/1073-7472.13.4.106

Park, M., Kjervik, D., Crandell, J., & Oermann, M.H. (2012). The relationship of ethics education to moral sensitivity and moral reasoning skills of nursing students. *Nursing Ethics, 19,* 568–580. doi:10.1177/0969733011433922

Peter, E., & Liaschenko, J. (2004). Perils of proximity: A spatiotemporal analysis of moral distress and moral ambiguity. *Nursing Inquiry, 11,* 218–225. doi:10.1111/j.1440-1800.2004.00236.x

Purtilo, R.B., & Doherty, R.F. (2011). *Ethical dimensions in the health professions* (5th ed.). St. Louis, MO: Elsevier Saunders.

Raines, M.L. (2000). Ethical decision making in nurses: Relationships among moral reasoning, coping style, and ethics stress. *JONA'S Healthcare Law, Ethics, and Regulation, 2,* 29–41. doi:10.1097/00128488-200002010-00006

Rodney, P., Doane, G.H., Storch, J., & Varcoe, C. (2006). Toward a safer moral climate. *Canadian Nurse, 102*(8), 24–27.

Rosenstand, N. (2006). *The moral of the story: An introduction to ethics* (5th ed.). New York, NY: McGraw-Hill.

Salyer, J., & Frazelle, M.R. (2014). Evolving and innovative opportunities for advanced practice nursing. In A.B. Hamric, J.A. Spross, & C.M. Hanson (Eds.), *Advanced practice nursing: An integrative approach* (5th ed., pp. 112–132). St. Louis, MO: Elsevier Saunders.

Schluter, J., Winch, S., Holzhauser, K., & Henderson, A. (2008). Nurse's moral sensitivity and hospital ethical climate: A literature review. *Nursing Ethics, 15*, 304–321. doi:10.1177/0969733007088357

Shumaker, S., Anderson, R., & Czajkowski, S. (1990). Psychological aspects of HRQOL measurement: Tests and scales. In B. Spilker (Ed.), *Quality of life assessments in clinical trials* (pp. 95–113). New York, NY: Raven Press.

Shuman, A.G., Montas, S.M., Barnosky, A.R., Smith, L.B., Fins, J.J., & McCabe, M.S. (2013). Clinical ethics consultation in oncology. *Journal of Oncology Practice, 9*, 240–245. doi:10.1200/JOP.2013.000901

Thiroux, J.P. (2001). *Ethics: Theory and practice* (7th ed.). Upper Saddle River, NJ: Prentice Hall.

Tishelman, C., Bernhardson, B.-M., Blomberg, K., Börjeson, S., Franklin, L., Johansson, E., … Ternestedt, B.-M. (2004). Issues and innovations in nursing practice: Complexity in caring for patients with advanced cancer. *Journal of Advanced Nursing, 45*, 420–429. doi:10.1046/j.1365-2648.2003.02925.x

Walker, M.U. (1993). Keeping moral space open. New images of ethics consulting. *Hastings Center Report, 23*(2), 33–40. doi:10.2307/3562818

Wright, D., & Brajtman, S. (2011). Relational and embodied knowing: Nursing ethics within the interprofessional team. *Nursing Ethics, 18*, 20–30. doi:10.1177/0969733010386165

Zuzelo, P.R. (2010). *The clinical nurse specialist handbook* (2nd ed.). Burlington, MA: Jones & Bartlett Learning.